The Complete

Atkins Diet

Guide

Ultimate Weight Loss Solution for a Healthy You

Sandra Baker

Contents

Introduction

The Atkins diet is based on a low-carb lifestyle and it is one of the most powerful weight-loss plans in the world. Avid followers of this dieting plan claim that this diet lets them lose weight while eating as much food as they want. It is a powerful weight-loss tool, but that statement is not entirely accurate. The golden rule of losing weight is that you must burn more calories than you consume. So when you are gauging the effectiveness of any dieting plan, then you need to keep that fact in mind. Will it help you remain at a calorie deficit? In regard to the Atkins diet, it will most definitely accomplish that goal.

There have been a lot of studies done that show low-carb diets can actually cause people to lose weight without the need for tracking calories. That tells me that it's easy to remain at a calorie deficit while consuming fewer carbs.

The Atkins diet was originally dismissed as unhealthy because of its focus on foods high in fat. Until recently, fats were considered to be unhealthy, but in reality the right fats are extremely healthy. In fact, even bad fats are harmless when you compare them to artificial sugars and other GMOs.

Since that important revelation, there has been an increase in the number of studies done on low-carb dieting. The results have been quite extraordinary. Lower blood sugar levels, higher HDL cholesterol counts, and significant weight loss are all found to be achievable under the Atkins diet.

The reason low-carb diets are so effective lies in the higher intake of fats and protein, both of which will reduce your overall appetite. You'll end up eating fewer calories without having to give it much thought. That's why people don't really have to count calories on this diet. However, I still encourage you to keep track of what you eat because it helps you boost the effectiveness of this diet.

The 4 Phases of the Atkins Diet

1. Introduction: During this phase of the diet, you will consume fewer than 20 grams in carbs every day. Your focus will be on high-fat, high-protein foods, along with vegetables.

2. Balancing: Now you will slowly add in a few nuts and a small amount of fruit to your diet. This ensures that you are getting the right nutrients while still restricting carbs.

3. Fine-Tuning: When your weight-loss goal is within reach, you will add more carbs into your diet until the weight loss starts to slow down.

4: Maintenance: By this point, you will be able to eat as many healthy carbs as you want, but you will need to keep track so that you do not start gaining weight back.

Introduction

Some people tend to follow the first phase indefinitely. This is known as the ketogenic diet, but for the purpose of this book we're going to walk through all four phases. For now, let's have a quick overview of some foods so that you have a basic understanding. Later, we will look at these foods in more detail.

Foods that you Should Avoid

➢ Foods with Refined Sugar – Soda, snack cakes, ice cream, etc.
➢ Grains – Bread, wheat, rye, rice, etc.
➢ Vegetable Oil – Soybean, corn, canola, etc.
➢ Trans Fat Foods – These are found in processed foods. Look for the word "hydrogenated" on the label.
➢ Low-Fat Foods – These are loaded with sugar and carbs.
➢ Starchy Vegetables – These are loaded with carbs. You want to avoid these during the introduction phase.
➢ Fruits – You will also want to avoid these during the introduction phase.
➢ Legumes – Beans and other legumes are all restricted during the introduction phase.

Foods that you Can Eat

➢ Meats – This is the best part of the Atkins diet. You can enjoy pretty much any meat, including bacon and pork!

- ➤ Seafood – Salmon and sardines are generally among the best.
- ➤ Eggs – These contain a ton of omega-3 fatty acids and are a staple of a low-carb diet.
- ➤ Low-Carb Vegetables – Kale, spinach, and broccoli.
- ➤ Full-Fat Dairy Products – You should always choose full-fat options when consuming dairy products. Milk is high in carbs so it should be avoided.
- ➤ Nuts and Seeds – Use these sparingly since they contain small amounts of carbs.
- ➤ Healthy Fat – Avocados are a super food and will boost the result of any low-carb diet. You can also use olive oil, coconut oil, and avocado oil.

Beverages that You Can Enjoy

- ➤ Water – You can drink as much water as you want.
- ➤ Coffee – Coffee is actually healthy as long as you don't overload it with cream and sugar.
- ➤ Green Tea – This is an extremely healthy beverage.
- ➤ Alcohol – Limit yourself to dry wines and avoid high-carb beverages like beer.

There are a lot of options that you can enjoy when you are following the Atkins diet. Foods that are considered fattening like bacon, heavy cream, and cheese are all perfectly okay. When you're on a low-carb diet, your body will start burning fat as energy and it will reduce your appetite. The result is that you can eat these foods while losing weight. Who would have ever thought that bacon could be a part of a healthy diet?

You'll Eventually Add in Healthy Carbs

Despite what many people believe, dieting does not have to be overly restrictive for it to be effective. The Atkins diet proves that with its flexibility. In fact, you will only be restricting carbs completely for two weeks before you start adding healthy ones back into your diet. This restrictive phase is known as the Introduction. Once you have made it through that two-week period, you will start adding in healthy carbs like fruits, potatoes, and berries.

However, even though you can add some carbs back into your diet, chances are that you might need to keep an eye on carbs for life since it will help keep the weight off. The Atkins diet is designed to help you find that sweet spot for the number of carbs required to maintain a steady weight.

Can Vegetarians Eat a Low-Carb Diet?

While it is possible to mix the Atkins diet with a vegetarian lifestyle, it is extremely difficult. You can replace meats with soy-based products as long as you add healthy oils to them for the added fat. It's worth noting that you need to consume more fat than protein on a low-carb diet.

Some vegetarians can eat dairy products, which would make it much easier since you can get your protein from eggs and your fats can come from butter and cheese.

Learning to Make Atkins-Friendly Snacks

Making healthy low-carb snacks is not as difficult as some people tend to believe. A lot of people agree that when they follow the Atkins diet, they experience a significant drop in their appetite. The reason is because when we train our body to start burning fat as energy, we will feel full for longer because we're actually using the fuel rather than storing it.

Most people are able to stick with a three-meals-per-day eating plan. In fact, you can mix this diet with intermittent fasting and live comfortably off of two meals per day.

If you do happen to get hungry in between meals though, it's essential that you eat a healthy snack rather than go hungry. This book will go into detail about making snacks that are Atkins friendly, but here are a few examples:

> - Hard-boiled egg
> - Leftover food from meals
> - Cheese
> - Dried meat
> - Palm full of nuts
> - Greek yogurt
> - Berries

> ➢ Fruit (only from Phase 2 forward)

Following the Atkins Diet at Restaurants

Following the Atkins diet is not that difficult when you decide to eat out. You just have to understand your food groups and which ones you are allowed at your specific phase of the plan. Here are some examples of a few small changes that you can make:

> ➢ Order an extra side of vegetables to replace bread, rice, or other high-carb food.
> ➢ Order fatty fish or another healthy meat as your main course.
> ➢ Order extra butter or olive oil with your meal.

The Atkins Diet Comes with Some Amazing Benefits

You are reading this book because you've heard just how powerful of a weight-loss tool that the Atkins diet can be, but there are a lot of other amazing benefits that are associated with this diet. Let's look at those benefits, starting with the obvious.

#1: You Will Lose Weight by Following the Atkins Diet

If you eat fewer carbs and stay at a calorie deficit, then you are going to lose weight, guaranteed! Some followers have seen drops of more than 100 pounds! The amount of weight you lose will depend on your adherence to the plan. But one thing is an absolute guarantee: if you restrict carbs, you will lose weight.

Low-carb dieting plans like the Atkins diet force your body to adapt by burning fat as fuel. Once this happens, it stops storing foods you eat. It will burn them immediately. Mix in an exercise routine and you'll experience even better results!

#2: It Will Improve the Health of Your Heart

We all know that obesity significantly increases your risk of heart disease, so lowering weight will positively affect the health of your heart. Furthermore, following a low-carb diet also reduces the risk of high blood pressure. When we consume carbs, our body will produce insulin that will hold onto excess fat for later use. Low-carb dieting will decrease the bad cholesterol while boosting the good cholesterol, effectively reducing blood pressure.

In short, we want our body to burn fat immediately rather than store it. Stored fat is like wax in your blood, eventually clogging arteries and forming blood clots.

#3: Lower Your Blood Sugar Levels

Increased blood sugar levels lead to both heart disease and obesity. In today's world of high-sugar foods and processed convenience, it should come as no surprise that most Americans have high blood sugar levels. Following the Atkins diet will help your body to process sugar correctly, lowering

Introduction

your risk of diseases like diabetes. In fact, individuals who are on insulin are sometimes able to slowly stop using it when they follow a low-carb lifestyle. Of course, you should never attempt this without approval from your doctor.

All carbs convert into sugar once consumed. In fact, eating two slices of whole wheat bread will spike your blood sugar level just as much as drinking a can of soda!

#4: Prevents Metabolic Syndrome
The Atkins diet can prevent metabolic syndrome. Abdominal obesity and elevated cholesterol can both be addressed through this amazing dietary strategy. Thanks to the healthy amount of protein you consume on this diet, you will also help preserve your muscle mass.

One of the problems with most diets is that they cause us to lose weight, but they also have the side effect of causing our muscle mass to drop. That causes our metabolism to dwindle to low levels so we feel exhausted all of the time. However, as your body adapts to burning fat as a primary source of energy, you'll start to experience a significant boost in energy. Plus your muscle mass will not suffer so you will experience a boost in your metabolic rate as a result.

#5: Atkins is Amazing at Controlling your Appetite
At first, you might have some cravings. This will be especially true during the introduction to the Atkins diet. When you

eliminate carbs, your body will start to go through carb withdrawal. You will crave sweets and sugars but it does not take much time for your body to adapt. Once it does, your cravings will be eliminated and you will start to experience a suppressed appetite.

If you find that you're struggling with cravings, then there are several tricks that you can use to help stave them off.

> ➤ Drink more water since most cravings come as a result of dehydration.
> ➤ Eat a healthy snack between meals.
> ➤ Identify emotional eating patterns and eliminate them.

As you start to live a healthier life, you will become familiar with your own body. That helps you identify triggers for food cravings and eliminate them.

#6: Experience an Improvement in Brain Function
One of the myths surrounding low-carb diets is that they will affect your brain function in a negative way. But the truth is that once your body has adapted to the lack of carbs, then the new metabolic process of using fat as the primary fuel source will actually lead to an improvement in brain function. Healthy fats and vitamin B are both essential to improved brain function and they are both found in foods that we'll focus on in the Atkins diet.

Berries, which are allowed in small quantities, are also proven to help your brain cells regenerate.

#7: Improves Physical Endurance
We know that the Atkins diet can help you lose weight, but when your body starts learning to metabolize fat, you will experience a boost in performance as well. That's because burning fat is like giving your body high octane fuel to burn. The metabolic increase that you'll experience is so significant that you will be able to push yourself further.

The boost in endurance is one of the reasons why athletes are swapping over to low-carb diets.

#8: Atkins Diet Promotes More Nutrients
By focusing on the foods that are allowed on the Atkins diet, you will be eating more nutrients than you're probably used to. These vitamins and minerals will impact your health in ways that you can't even imagine. You'll feel so much better and have much more energy to tackle your everyday life. When you eat a healthy meal, you will feel amazing afterwards, whereas when you eat meals like pizza, you feel bloated and tired afterwards.

Meals on the Atkins diet will include a sizeable portion of protein and fatty food, along with a large helping of vegetables.

#9: Atkins Dieting will Decrease Inflammation
Inflammation is a defensive mechanism in the body that happens when we are injured or sick. Even healthy people experience a certain amount of inflammation. The problem is that the Western diet is so bad that it leads to chronic inflammation. This can lead to serious health issues and diseases.

Insulin spikes contribute to chronic inflammation, so when you are able to get your blood sugar levels under control you'll prevent this from happening.

#10: Atkins Dieting Targets Abdominal Fat
Belly fat is one of the most dangerous types of fat because it impacts almost every organ in your body. It also produces the most harmful chemicals and hormones. Belly fat is shown to increase the risk of diabetes and cancer.

Low-carb dieting will target this fat first and you'll see it start to quickly fade. This is usually the most difficult fat to shed, but the Atkins diet will give you results that you can start to see within just a few weeks!

Are You Ready?
If you are serious about losing weight, then the Atkins diet can be an amazing tool to help you on your journey. This book will help you get started on your journey. I can show you every step to take, but you are the only one who can motivate

yourself to keep at it. I warn you that, in the beginning, it's going to take some getting used to. You might feel sluggish as your body adapts to using fat as a source of fuel.

At the end of the day, this lifestyle is an extremely effective way to lose weight. You are in for an amazing journey!

Chapter 1
The Atkins Diet Explained

Why is it that low-carb diets are so effective at helping people achieve their weight loss goals? There are actually quite a few scientific facts surrounding these amazing results. In fact, most people are surprised to learn that people who follow low-carb diets lose twice as much weight as those who follow traditional diets. Yet, so many people still scream at us to follow those traditional low-fat diets.

What makes it even more amazing is that a large chunk of this fat is taken away from the belly, which is the most dangerous type of fat. Plus the Atkins diet has the added bonus of providing you with a significant metabolic boost. Naturally, when you remove sugars from your diet then you will also reduce your risk of diabetes.

With that being said, there is some controversy surrounding low-carb diets, mainly having to do with the actual biology happening in our bodies. This chapter is going to walk you through some of the explanations to show you why the Atkins diet works and the science behind it.

Restricting Carbs Will Lower Insulin Levels

There's no controversy here. It's a well-known fact that when we reduce the amount of carbs we are consuming, then our liver does not have to produce as much insulin. Insulin is the main hormone that is used by the body to process glycogen and regulate our blood sugar levels.

Insulin directs our fat cells to produce and store more fat. So the higher level of insulin, the more weight we will gain. Then it will tell our body to burn sugar as energy instead of burning fat. In short, insulin will cause our body to store fat rather than burn it as energy.

Low-carb diets like the Atkins diet will lead to almost immediate drops in insulin production. In fact, this is the main reason behind the effectiveness of low-carb diets. When the body starts burning fat as energy, we feel better and are much healthier as a result.

The bottom line here is that lower insulin levels and weight loss are directly linked. The Atkins diet will lower your blood sugar levels and make sure that you are able to burn more fat.

Your Water Weight will Drop Rapidly
Individuals who start their journey on a low-carb diet tend to lose a large amount of weight in the beginning. That's because you will start rapidly losing water weight almost instantly! The reasoning behind this is in two parts:

For starters, the lower insulin levels free up the kidneys to start filtering and removing excess sodium from our body. This also has the added bonus of lowering our blood pressure.

Glycogen is how the body stores carbs. The problem with glycogen is that it is bonded by water. So when we reduce our carb intake, we do not have to store as much water. Therefore, that extra water is shed.

Neither of those things happens on any other diet, even if you were to significantly reduce calorie intake. Water weight will remain the same.

The problem is that some people tend to argue that the weight lost on a low-carb diet is only water weight, but that is clearly not the case. This is just an added advantage but the majority of weight lost comes in the form of fat being burned.

Atkins Dieting is Loaded with Protein

Individuals who adopt a low-carb lifestyle will end up eating more protein because they are replacing grains with foods that are high in protein. The amazing thing about protein is that it reduces appetite, boosts metabolism, and helps increase your muscle mass so that you are able to burn more calories.

In fact, many advocates of the Atkins diet believe that this is the main factor in its effectiveness. The fact is that a low-carb lifestyle will naturally lead to higher protein consumption. Therefore, you will experience a significant reduction in appetite and a boost in your metabolism. This is the opposite of the effect that calorie restrictive diets have on the body.

Atkins Dieting Comes with a Metabolic Advantage

Although there are a lot of reasons why a low-carb diet is extremely effective, I feel that one of the most advantageous factors is that it puts you at a metabolic advantage. Some people believe that it's the higher protein intake that leads to this higher metabolic rate, but the fact remains that, whatever the case, low-carb diets like the Atkins diet will have this effect.

When our carb intake is exceptionally low, the body will start converting protein into glucose. This will essentially waste a lot of calories in the beginning, but it's a temporary loss because the body will quickly adapt. Ketones will be formed in the body and replace that process as a primary source of fuel after just a few days. That's when you will experience a significant boost in energy, and you will start rapidly losing weight when that happens.

The Atkins diet will give you at an advantage.

Atkins Dieting is Lower in Food Rewards

One sacrifice that you will have to make is with your selection of foods. At first, the Atkins diet is going to be quite restrictive and, while that does change, removing sugars and processed foods from your diet is not an easy change. But I promise you that once you transition, you'll feel so amazing that you'll never want to go back.

The selection of foods that you are allowed to eat is reduced. Wheat and sugar are two cornerstones of the Western diet so giving them up is a noticeable change. I won't lie and say that it's easy. Nor will I say that it's unnoticeable. But the results will be well worth the effort!

The problem is that those unhealthy choices are highly rewarding so we end up overeating. Once you get used to healthy foods though, they will become even more rewarding.

Atkins Dieting Reduces your Appetite

A reduction in appetite will lead to an automatic reduction in calorie intake, which will ultimately lead to weight loss. Remember that the only way to lose weight is to consume fewer calories than you burn. This is another reason that a low-carb diet is so effective. In fact, most experts agree that this is the main reason behind the success of the Atkins diet.

Even so, low-carb dieters still experience greater weight loss than traditional dieters who restrict carbs. In addition to a decrease in appetite, ketosis also boosts you metabolic rate so you'll burn more calories. That is the science behind Atkins dieting's enhanced weight loss potential.

Atkins Dieting for the Long Term

One of the essential elements of losing weight is that you must have a system in place so that you can keep the weight off. So many people fall into the trap of losing weight for a short amount of time, only to watch themselves gain it back. The reason is because they stop following the habits that led to weight loss in the first place.

Atkins dieting is designed to help you lose weight and then find a healthy balance in the end. You will be opening yourself back up to healthy carbs and restricting fewer foods. That's why this lifestyle has the potential for long-term success. You are essentially customizing habits that will be easy to follow in the long term.

There are always going to be naysayers who claim that low-carb diets are unhealthy and that we must follow the food pyramid – a chart created before we truly understood the human body and how foods affect it. Do not let these people distract you from your goals.

The Atkins diet works on both sides of the calorie weight loss equation. It lowers your appetite so your intake is reduced while also boosting your metabolic rate so you burn more calories.

Make no mistake though. Calories still count, but a low-carb lifestyle will help keep those calories under control!

Chapter 2
Atkins Diet Food Guide

In the beginning phase, the Atkins diet is quite restrictive in favor of loosening up as you get close to achieving your weight-loss goals. What can you eat for breakfast to replace those pancakes in the beginning? What can you add to meals to replace pasta and bread?

While it might be restrictive, the Atkins diet has the potential to create some amazing meals and gives you access to amazing food. I mean, what other diet allows you to eat bacon and still lose weight?

This chapter is going to show you some of the foods that you can enjoy while starting your journey on the Atkins diet. I'm also going to show you some of the foods that you should avoid. Low carb doesn't have to be overly complicated. In fact, I am going to make it really simple for you.

Low-Carb List of Foods to Enjoy

Meat: You can eat any type of meat you want. Just be sure to avoid cured meats that contain added sugar. When eating chicken, you should also eat the skin when possible because it's the fattiest part. Stick to organic grass-fed options if your budget allows. Organic foods are always better, but it's better to be 90% compliant than not at all, so if you can't afford these organic meats, then stick to standard ones.

Fish and Seafood: Fatty fish like salmon and mackerel are the best choices, but you are allowed to eat any foods that come from the ocean. Fish is one of the most brain-healthy foods on the planet.

Eggs: Eggs are one of the staples of low-carb dieting. You'll find yourself eating these quite often. Again, you should choose organic eggs if your budget allows.

High-Fat Sauces: Butter and cream are both important parts of a low-carb diet. You'll find yourself going out of your way to add fat to meals. The amazing thing about fatty sauces is that they add flavor to your foods. You can add all of the butter and olive oil you want!

Vegetables: You can eat any vegetable that grows above the ground but you need to avoid those that are underground. Just pay attention to the carb count of vegetables that you are eating. Also, remember that for the purpose of low-carb dieting, fiber does not count against your daily total since your body does not process it.

Dairy Products: Be very careful here because some dairy products contain sugar. Full-fat options are always going to be the best bet for Atkins diet followers. Cheese and sour cream are amazing ways to fuel your metabolism, while milk is best avoided due to its high sugar count.

Nuts and Seeds: You should use these as a snack in the place of popcorn or chips. Be careful because these do contain carbs so you have to eat them sparingly. It's best to avoid them altogether during the Introduction phase but if you have a craving, then you can snack on them.

Berries: This is another food that you will introduce to your diet during Phase 2. Berries provide a significant metabolic boost. They are also an amazing snack that you can enjoy with whipped cream.

Low-Carb Beverages

Water: Water is an important part of a healthy lifestyle so be sure that you are drinking enough of it every day. You can also drink flavored sparkling water too!

Coffee: You can drink black coffee with a small amount of milk or cream. You are even allowed to add artificial sweetener so there is no reason to give up coffee altogether. In fact, you can use coconut oil and butter to create "bulletproof coffee."

Diet Drinks: Here is an area of controversy so let me clear it up right now. Zero-calorie beverages like Diet Coke do not count as carbs, so you can drink one or two of these per day. The problem is that they make you have sugar cravings. My recommendation is that you limit these to only a few servings per week at most.

Alcohol: Hard liquors are preferable over beer. In either case, consuming alcohol should be restricted during the Introduction phase and then limited to special occasions the rest of the time.

Dark Chocolate: You can look at the label to make sure that the dark chocolate you're eating has a low carb count. You are actually allowed to eat this type of snack and it's even used in a number of fat bombs.

Avoid all High-Carb Foods

Avoid Sugar: Soft drinks, candy, baked goods, and fruit juice are all horrible on your body, and you will have to completely eliminate these from your life. There are just so many healthy alternatives that, over time, you won't even miss these foods.

Grains: You have to avoid these altogether during the Introduction phase and then you'll slowly add whole grains back into your diet. However, you still want to limit them. Furthermore, there are some fantastic low-carb alternatives to these products.

Beans and Lentils: These are healthy foods, but they are loaded with carbs so you will need to avoid them during the

Introduction phase. However, this is one of the food sets that you can add back to your diet later.

Beer: You will need to avoid beer altogether since it's loaded with carbs. There are some low-carb beers available now so you can try these, but I still recommend that you limit your consumption of beer.

Fruit: This is another healthy food that is high in carbs. You'll have to avoid it during the Introduction phase and slowly add in fruit to your diet during the later phases.

Pay Close Attention to These Foods

Low-fat or fat-free products are usually unhealthy. Always read the labels for these products carefully. Sometimes these products might even prevent weight loss and they simply don't work. I have found that any foods created by humans to be "healthy" are usually not healthy at all. The true solution lies in natural foods. For instance, some of these foods will be loaded in sugar alcohol that will cause your body to react as if you have eaten carbs. The problem is that they still technically count as zero carbs, so it's well hidden on the food label.

So many companies out there will try to trick you with their "low-fat" junk food but a lot of these are loaded with sugar alcohol and sweeteners. In fact, one company was fined for blatantly lying about the carb content of their product.

There are two rules that you should always follow to avoid bad food choices:

1. Do not eat low-carb versions of cookies, candy bars, or other junk food. The only way you can break this rule is if you make the snack yourself and are 100% sure about the ingredients.
2. When you see a product that uses the words "net carbs" on the label, then the company is probably trying to legally fool you. These foods are rarely healthy choices.

While we encourage butter on the Atkins diet, you should definitely avoid margarine because it's made of unhealthy vegetable oils. Real butter tastes so much better and is quite healthy.

Keep it Real

Avoid processed foods. Always shop the outside of the supermarket since that's where the real foods are kept. Whole foods are so much better for you and you'll quickly find that your body responds much better to them.

One rule of thumb is to stick mostly to foods that would have been available a thousand years ago. If the food has a ton of ingredients on the label, then it's processed.

Lowering Carb Intake

How many grams of carbs should you eat on any given day? The standard Western diet usually means that people are consuming 300 grams of carbs per day, mostly in the form of harmful sugar. What we have discovered is when the average person can drop their daily carb intake to 100 grams, they will lose weight. The reason is because this means they would be giving up sugars and other super unhealthy junk food.

With the Atkins diet, our end goal will be somewhere around 100 grams per day, but we will need to restrict them even further in the beginning. The reason is that we want to show our body just how well it thrives when burning fat as energy. As you slowly move back into the normal range, then your metabolic rate will continue to burn high.

Low-carb diets usually restrict carbs to 20 grams per day, but they never show you a way to increase that count over time. It would be extremely difficult to maintain that lifestyle for the long term. Our main goal is going to be getting away from all of those unhealthy choices. We'll be paying more attention to the foods that go into our body.

Chapter 3
Healthy Atkins Diet Snacking

One of the main advantages of a low-carb diet is that it has powerful appetite suppression potential. But there will be days when you have a sudden hunger craving, so it's important to plan ahead for these times. We are vulnerable when we're hungry so it's essential that you have snacks ready for these moments. When you are hungry, eat. Any diet that requires you to go hungry is going to fail.

Fortunately, there are a number of amazing snack choices for us as we continue on the Atkins diet. Cravings can lead to fatigue and lapses in concentration. Plus it causes us to overeat during our next meal. I am going to show you a few snacks that are friendly to the Atkins diet and that can be prepared in mere minutes. To make this easier, I'll separate these snacks into two separate phases.

Snacks for the Introduction Phase
- ➢ 1 oz. string cheese
- ➢ Celery with cream cheese
- ➢ Cucumber stuffed with tuna salad
- ➢ 5 olives, green or black. You can even stuff them with cheese.
- ➢ Half an avocado
- ➢ Beef jerky (be careful not to eat too much)

- ➢ Deviled egg
- ➢ Cheddar cheese wrapped in lettuce
- ➢ Green beans wrapped in sliced ham (not cured in sugar)

Snacks for Ongoing Weight Loss

- ➢ 1/2 cup of unsweetened whole yogurt. You can mix in coconut or another berry/fruit.
- ➢ Celery sticks with peanut butter
- ➢ Cucumber stuffed with ricotta
- ➢ 2 melon chunks wrapped in either ham or salmon
- ➢ Fruit/cheese kebabs
- ➢ Scoop of cottage cheese topped with salsa
- ➢ 4 oz. tomato juice and 1 tbsp. sour cream mixed together. Top this mixture with avocado chunks.
- ➢ Blueberries and string cheese
- ➢ 1 piece of fruit (last two phases only)
- ➢ Hummus with low-carb, crispy bread (Phase 4 only)

Fat Bombs Are an Amazing Atkins Dieting Snack

Fat bombs are an amazing high-fat dessert snack that will actually give your metabolism a huge boost and help you melt away fat! These are great for those of you who have a sweet tooth and need a daily dose of sweetness. Ketogenic fat bombs will solve these cravings in a single bite!

Always remember that for ketosis to take effect, your foods should be comprised of at least 75% healthy fat. That's why fat bombs are so amazing. They are loaded with fat so once you have gotten your body into ketosis, this boost of fat will provide you with a huge metabolic boost. In fact, I highly recommend that you eat a fat bomb every day about two hours after lunch.

For those of you who are not familiar with fat bombs, they are small, bite-sized snacks that are loaded with healthy fat. They usually contain about 85% fat. Since they contain so much fat, a single bite will satisfy your hunger for hours. Plus they give you a huge boost of energy.

Now let's look at actually making fat bombs. It's super easy. You just blend together all ingredients and then pour this mixture into a mold like a muffin tin or cupcake liner. Then place in the refrigerator or freezer until they harden. They will melt quickly since they are made of fat so you must keep them chilled until you're ready to eat them.

Fat bombs use three key ingredients:

➢ **Fat Base** – Coconut oil, butter, cream cheese, etc.
➢ **Flavor** – cocoa powder, spices, etc.
➢ **Mix-In** – Almonds, seeds, coconut, etc.

Coconut oil is the healthiest type of fat you can use for fat bombs. Your body does not store fat from coconut oil. It uses it immediately! Furthermore, it can last up to two years without going bad. It also gives your fat bombs a buttery flavor.

MCT oil is another amazing type of fat. It ignites your metabolism, giving you a quick and lasting boost of energy! In fact, MCT oil can provide you with energy through the entire day without crashing.

Stevia is the best flavor to use since it comes with no unpleasant aftertaste and is very healthy.

Fat bomb molds are a great tool for making preparation easy. You can even buy these molds in different shapes and sizes, including heart- and star-shaped designs. With this all in mind, here are a few easy-to-prepare fat bomb recipes.

Vanilla Coconut Bars

Ingredients

- ✓ 1 cup shredded coconut (unsweetened)
- ✓ 1/4 cup water
- ✓ 2 drops liquid stevia
- ✓ 2 tbsp. coconut oil
- ✓ 1/2 tsp. vanilla extract
- ✓ Dash of salt (about 1/8 tsp.)

Directions

1. Mix together all ingredients using a food processor. Press this mixture evenly into molds.

2. Place mold into the refrigerator for at least one hour before serving.

Nutrition

Calories: 138

Fat: 13g
Carbs: 4g
Protein: 1g
Fiber: 2g
Servings: 6

Walnut Nutter Butter Bombs

Ingredients

- ✓ 4 tbsp. butter
- ✓ 1/2 cup almond butter
- ✓ 1/2 cup coconut oil
- ✓ 6 drops liquid Stevia
- ✓ 2 tbsp. Chopped walnuts
- ✓ Dash of sea salt
- ✓ 1 bar dark chocolate, melted

Directions

1. Mix together all ingredients into a bowl and heat in microwave for approximately 30 seconds.

2. Whisk mixture until it's blended together.

3. Pour evenly into molds. Place in freezer for approximately 1 hour.

Nutrition
Calories: 138

Fat: 29g
Carbs: 3g
Protein: 3g
Fiber: 2g
Servings: 8

Stuffed Pecan Fat Bombs

Ingredients

- ✓ 8 pecans, halved
- ✓ 1/2 tsp. butter
- ✓ 1 ounce cream cheese
- ✓ Dash of sea salt

Directions

1. Roast pecans in oven at 350 degrees for approximately 10 minutes. Allow them to cool.

2. Mix together butter and cream cheese. It will be smooth and creamy.

3. Spread mixture between two pecan halves. Place in refrigerator.

Nutrition
Calories: 150
Fat: 31g

Carbs: 2g
Protein: 11g
Fiber: 1.2g
Servings: 4

Chocolate Peanut Butter Coconut Bombs

Ingredients

- ✓ 3/4 cup coconut oil
- ✓ 1/4 cup cocoa powder
- ✓ 1/4 cup natural unsweetened peanut butter
- ✓ 3 drops liquid stevia

Directions

1. Heat coconut oil in microwave until it melts. Divide this mixture into three separate bowls.

2. In one bowl, mix in cocoa powder until it's dissolved. Add 1 drop of liquid stevia.

3. In the second bowl, mix in peanut butter and blend until it's smooth. Add a drop of stevia.

4. In the final bowl, add 1 drop of stevia.

. Add the chocolate mixture evenly to molds and place in refrigerator for 10 minutes. Then spread peanut butter mixture on top of chocolate layers. Then refrigerate for 10 more minutes. Finally, spread the rest of the mixture over the top of each fat bomb. Chill for one hour.

Nutrition
Calories: 184
Fat: 20g
Carbs: 2g
Protein: 2g
Fiber: 1g
Servings: 10

Chapter 4
Set Goals and Track Them

Setting goals is one of the major factors in whether you are going to be successful and whether you are going to fail. Having the right goals in place will help you in so many ways. It is also a proven fact that people who put goals in place are twice as likely to achieve their dreams over those who try without goals. Think of it like a roadmap. If you are going on a trip, then you need a roadmap to help guide you along the way. Following the Atkins diet is a journey, and goals will help guide you all the way to the final destination – success!

With that said, setting bad goals will have the opposite effect. It will actually undermine your efforts and lead to frustration. This chapter is going to show you some of the benefits of setting the right goals and then walk you through the entire process so that you're setting the right ones. Are you ready to start setting goals that will change your life?

Setting Weight Loss Goals Has Some Amazing Benefits
Being able to set the right goals will lead to some amazing benefits. Even if you fail at a couple of goals, you are going to learn from those setbacks and move forward; whereas when you fail with no goals in place, you are likely to get frustrated and give up.

Goals Provide Direction

The biggest benefit of setting goals is that they give you a sense of direction. By knowing your destination, it's easier to find the easiest path to success. This is especially important when things get tough. Starting with a lifetime goal of being healthy is great, but the goals you need to focus on are the smaller, more achievable milestones along the way. Rather than wandering aimlessly from one point to the next, having a single direction makes it much easier to reach the end.

Put Your Focus on What's Important

Goals will provide a clear focus on your desired results. It shows you what's important and gives you something to focus on. You will need to really think about what it is that you are trying to achieve. Weight loss alone is usually not enough. Why are you trying to lose weight? Is it so that you look better? Are you trying to keep from feeling sluggish in the afternoon? Understanding what is important to you helps keep you motivated. The main reason so many people do not achieve their goals is because they do not define what's important. Highly successful people are laser focused. They set clear, measurable goals and then work hard to achieve them.

Helps You Make Better Decisions

As we just saw, setting the right goals will help you focus on what's important, which leads to making better decisions regarding your health. When you know exactly what you want to accomplish, you will be able to map out most of the steps. This will make it much easier to make important decisions. In fact, most decisions will be made while you are laying out your overall plan. After that, all you will need to do is make adjustments.

Goals Put You in the Driver's Seat
Take control of your health by setting important goals. Without having goals in place, you are essentially just going along for the ride. You will never be in full control of your life until you have set goals. You do not want to just wander around aimlessly hoping for the best. This one benefit will put you in full control of whether you succeed or fail.

Having Goals Keeps you Motivated
One of the most amazing things about being focused on a goal is that it keeps you motivated. When we can actually see our accomplishments, we tend be more successful. This is especially important when things get tough. As you work towards achieving your long-term goal, you'll achieve some of your short-term goals as well. Success has a snowball effect in that it builds momentum. As you achieve small goals, the next one becomes easier. Being motivated makes it much easier to work through the most difficult times.

Set Yourself Up for Success by Setting the Right Goals
Now that we have gone through the benefits of setting goals, it's time to start setting the right goals. One mistake that I see

so many people make is that they establish poor goals that set them up for failure. Don't be one of those people. Here's a step-by-step look at setting goals that will set you up for success.

Step 1: Focus on Process-Oriented Goals
Setting weight loss goals should focus on the process rather than on the outcome. Outcome goals are set with a focus on the end result. In other words, setting a goal of losing 10 pounds is a goal that focuses on the outcome. While this is not necessarily a bad goal, it does not really show you how to achieve that end.

Rather than saying that you want to lose 10 pounds, you would create a goal that is based on the process. For the Atkins diet, a good process goal would be to reduce your carb intake down to no more than 20 grams per day. We're actually going to lay out a very detailed plan later.

Process goals are the best way to set yourself up for success when it comes to weight loss because they focus more on changing your habits. These changes will make it easier to lose weight.

Step 2: Set SMART Goals
SMART is an acronym that we will be using to set ourselves up for success. When setting your process goals, be sure that they meet the following checklist criteria.

Set Goals and Track Them

Specific – Goals absolutely must be specific. Broad or vague goals can be disastrous. For instance, a goal to "exercise more" is not going to help. Instead, you would want to set a goal like "walk for 30 minutes every day" because this is more specific. You are making a declaration as to what you will be doing and how long you'll be doing it. Another specific goal could be: "I'm going to spend two weeks restricting carbs completely and then record my progress."

Measurable – Being able to measure goals is essential to determining how successful you are. If you can't measure a goal, then you have no way of tracking your progress. "Eating healthier" is not exactly measurable but "restricting calorie intake to 2,000 calories per day" is measurable.

Attainable – This one is extremely important and it's also where most people tend to mess up. Your goals must be attainable and realistic. Setting goals that are impossible to achieve sets you up for failure. Restricting your carb intake to 20 grams per day is an attainable goal.

Relevant – Your goals must be relevant to your weight-loss goals. Never set goals that other people want you to obtain. Set goals based on what's important to you. Is weight loss your primary goal? Maybe you're just looking to lower your risk of heart disease. Whatever the case, make sure that you are setting goals based on your happiness.

Time-Limited – Setting deadlines has a powerful effect on how we perceive a goal. If we're restricting carbs to 20 grams per day, then circle a day on the calendar to check in on your progress. Time limits have a way of motivating us because we have used them our entire lives.

Step 3: Set Long-Term and Short-Term Goals
Long-term goals will help you see the bigger picture. They will shift your train of thought towards your overall goals. For instance, the Atkins diet is designed to swap all of your unhealthy carbs for healthy ones. This is a long-term process goal that requires several steps. As with all long-term goals, we will be setting short-term goals as steps towards achieving this overall goal. Here's a quick example:

Long-Term Goal – Lose 30 pounds in 6 months by transitioning my diet to healthy carbs.

Short-Term Goal 1 – Restrict carbs to 20 grams per day for one month.

Short-Term Goal 2 – Add fruits back into my diet. No more than 1 serving of fruit per day. Try not get over 50 grams of carbs per day.

Short-Term Goal 3 – Add all healthy carbs back into my diet. Stay away from sugar and processed foods.

Short-Term Goal 4 – Keep a close eye on my weight to make sure it stays steady.

Step 4: Plan for Setbacks
Setbacks are going to happen when making lifestyle changes. Those who are successful are the ones that plan for these setbacks rather than submitting to them. It's much better to plan ahead for the day when they happen. Identify potential roadblocks. Most dieting setbacks come in the form of holidays, barbeques, and family reunions. Go ahead and plan for those instances now. What will you do during the holidays? Will you give yourself a cheat day or will you just stick to the low-carb selections available?

Step 5: Set Aside Time for Assessment and Make Adjustments
I recommend that you set aside time every month to assess your goals. You might need to make adjustments to your overall plan. If you are on track, then you will be even more motivated to continue. Success begets success, but you have to take the time to acknowledge it.

Goals are the foundation to making lasting change. They are going to mean the difference between whether you succeed or whether you fail.

Chapter 5
Step-by-Step Guide to Following the Atkins Diet

By this point, we have all of the basics out of the way so now it's time to get started on this fantastic new lifestyle! The Atkins diet is one of the most fantastic ways of improving your health. You will literally watch the pounds melt away as you build up better habits. So we're going to start with a few tips that you should always keep in the back of your mind and then move on to an actual step-by-step guide to getting started.

Atkins Diet Tips You Must Follow

As we mentioned earlier in this book, you must set goals in order to have a chance of being successful. Individuals who set goals are twice as likely to achieve their vision. Healthy, achievable goals are going to be an important part of your journey into this new lifestyle.

It's important that you understand exactly how the Atkins diet works. Fortunately, that's why you are reading this book. Committing to any new lifestyle requires a commitment, but the only way we can fully commit to something is by understanding it. The Atkins diet is broken down into four phases, each one with its own set of goals. The idea is to clean up your diet so that you end up with healthier eating habits.

Another valuable tip is to constantly surround yourself with motivation, especially when you're starting on your journey. Join some communities and stay active. Share your goals with others so that you're being held accountable. Losing weight is so much easier when you are having fun and being active with other people.

Become familiar with the foods that you are allowed to eat. This will change during the course of the diet but you have to understand what types of foods are high in carbs and which ones are not. While it's certainly okay to memorize a list in the beginning, the only way you will master the Atkins diet is to fully understand what you're putting into your body.

Make sure that you drink enough water. Divide your weight in half. That's the amount of water (in ounces) that you should be drinking every day. You do not count coffee and tea as part of your water for the day. Staying hydrated is essential to losing weight. One of the problems that we all have is that we're dehydrated. When we're dehydrated, we will start to crave food and have a severe lack of energy. Furthermore, your body will drop a lot of water weight during Phase 1 of the Atkins diet so it's easy to get dehydrated.

Do not restrict fats. You will not lose weight on the Atkins diet unless you eat a lot of fat. I know that is the opposite of traditional dieting, but the more fat you consume, the more weight you will lose. Think of fat like fuel that lights your metabolism. The more fuel you add, the hotter it burns. Healthy fats are quite beneficial too. They help your body absorb vitamins and minerals.

Always eat when you're hungry. Again, this is the opposite of what some people believe when it comes to dieting. They think that it's healthy to be hungry. You just need to have the willpower to be successful. That is the belief. However, the fact is that biology will always win in a battle against willpower. Eventually, you will give in to your cravings so it's better to just eat when you're hungry. Have a selection of low-carb snacks ready so that when you are hungry, you have something to eat.

Making smarter choices is always going to get you further than trying to beat willpower. With that being said, it's time we move deeper into the journey towards a healthier lifestyle.

Step 1: The Introduction Phase

Now we're going to take a close look at each phase of the Atkins diet. You will need to jumpstart your weight loss so Phase 1 is going to phase out all carbs in favor of foods that are high in healthy fat. If you have read anything about the ketogenic diet, then you will be familiar with this phase. The problem is that most people will simply try to stay in this phase indefinitely, but removing carbs forever is not a sustainable long-term goal. This is just the key to jumpstarting your metabolic burn! You will learn how to follow healthier habits while removing some of the worst foods from your diet. It is also during this phase that you will lose the most weight.

Our goal is going to be to first remove carbs completely from our diet and then slowly replace them with healthier choices. We want to learn the exact number of carbs that we can consume to continue losing weight. This is known as a personal carb balance and it's the ultimate goal of the Atkins diet.

This step is all about changing the way your body operates. We do this by developing healthier habits, which means we have to be strict in the beginning. Just remember that you will not have to remain this strict forever. The length of this introduction phase is going to be dependent on the goals you have set for yourself. It can last anywhere from 2 weeks to 2 months. You will stay in this phase until you are approximately 15 pounds from your weight goal.

Carb crash is a very real thing!

A lot of people who start out on a low-carb diet experience carb crash after a few days. This happens when the body uses up all of its glucose reserves and it has not gotten used to burning fat as a primary source of energy. Some symptoms will include jitters, shaking, fatigue, and irritability. It's important that you understand this is temporary. It will only last for a day or two. Once your body starts burning fat as a primary source of energy, you'll have more energy and feel much better than you did before you started this journey.

If this crash gets too bad, then eat a piece of low-carb fruit. This will help balance out the body but it won't throw you out of ketosis. The goal is to be restrictive during the introduction, but it's better to be a little lenient rather than feel awful. Just remember that you cannot use this as an excuse to overload on carbs. Eat a piece of fruit and then wait for the symptoms to subside.

Another way that you can avoid carb crashing is by having a cup of bouillon every day for the first week. Sometimes the lower sodium levels are responsible for these symptoms so the bouillon will help.

During this phase, you will start to lose weight at a rapid level. That's why it's such a powerful diet. Once you start getting close to your target weight, the loss will start to balance itself out. You will quickly find that as your body starts burning fat as a primary source of energy, at that point, you will experience a significant boost in energy. You'll feel amazing and will be much more productive.

It's essential that you drop your daily carb intake to 20 grams when on this phase. You cannot go over that amount if you want to melt away that weight. Although the Atkins diet is restrictive in the early phases, it becomes much more lenient as we move closer to our goal. This will be the most difficult step though.

Final Tips for Step 1

➢ Clear out your refrigerator, freezer, and pantry. Remove foods that are high in carbs and replace them with low-carb alternatives.

➢ Consider keeping a food journal to track what goes into your body. This helps you identify patterns.

➢ Never, ever allow yourself to go hungry.

➢ Prepare snacks and have them readily available for cravings.

➢ Remember that fiber does not count toward your carb count.

Step 2: Transition from Phase 1 to Phase 2

You should check your weight every two weeks and then decide whether you are going to stay in Phase 1 or move on to Phase 2. Remember, you want to be within 15 pounds of your weight goal before making the transition. You'll lose the most weight during Phase 1 so make sure you're okay with moving on.

This step of the Atkins journey is where we start balancing our diet. While we might have stayed away from nuts in the previous step, it's time to start adding them into our diet because they are one of the most metabolic-friendly snacks on the planet!

Let's make this super easy by adding nuts back to our list of approved foods. You can add in 3 grams of carbs in the form of nuts and seeds per day. Here's a quick look at some examples of 3 grams' worth of nuts or seeds:

➢ 30 almonds
➢ 3 tbsp. macadamia nuts
➢ 2 tbsp. peanut butter
➢ 2 tbsp. pistachios
➢ 4 tbsp. sunflower seeds, shelled
➢ 24 walnut halves

I recommend that you portion these servings out ahead of time so that you don't risk overeating. Buy some small baggies and add a serving of nuts to each one so that you can quickly grab it and snack on it.

Keep in mind that this phase is where we start transitioning into a permanent new lifestyle. We're going to be introducing some carbs back into our diet. That means our daily carb intake will also need to be raised gradually.

Balancing carbs is the key to long-term success. We want to remove all of those wasteful carbs found in sugars and processed foods. We'll be replacing them with fruits, vegetables, and other healthy choices.

Add in carbs at 5-gram increments every three days. You will need to pay close attention to the carbs you eat though. Identify any that might lead to cravings or cause you to feel sluggish. Avoid those foods and find the ones you can thrive on. This will be different for everyone so it's important that you pay close attention to your body. It will look something like this:

Days 1-3: 25 grams of carbs daily.

Days 4-6: 30 grams of carbs daily.

Days 7-9: 35 grams of carbs daily.

Stop at around 35 grams of carbs per day and give it a couple of weeks to see if you continue to lose weight.

You will want to keep an eye on your weight as you gradually add carbs back to your diet. Remember, this does not give you license to eat a bunch of snack cakes and sugary treats. The carbs you consume should be obtained from healthy sources.

Here is a look at some of the carbs you can add back into your diet:

➢ Nut and seeds
➢ Berries

- ➢ Melon
- ➢ Cherries
- ➢ Greek yogurt

If you are still losing weight at 35 grams after two weeks, then you can gradually move your way up to 50 grams per day. Again, raise your carb allowance by 5 grams every 3 days until you're at 50. Now you can start adding vegetable juices and legumes into your diet.

Phase 2 of the Atkins diet is all about learning your personal carb tolerance. This is the key to long-term weight loss.

Step 3: Maintain your Weight After Dieting

By this point, you will be extremely close to achieving your weight loss goal. I'm sure you're excited but there is also a voice inside that is worried about falling off the wagon. Don't worry. Everyone who makes a lifestyle change experiences that same voice. What we have to do is make long-term success as simple as possible. We do that by finding what works right for our unique life.

We're going to keep gradually raising our carb allowance until we settle at a final amount. These are the final rungs on the ladder to a healthier life.

You will continue on Phase 3 until you have achieved your desired weight and have kept it off for at least one month.

Step-by-Step Guide

You'll need to gradually adjust your carb allowance until you are at the perfect amount. This is all about getting it to the perfect point, which will be different for everyone. Think of this as the dress rehearsal for your new lifestyle.

Everyone has a different personal carb balance.

You can only find this amount by slowly raising your allowance until you stop losing weight. Here's the easiest way to accomplish this end.

1. When you stop losing weight, lower your carb allowance by 10 grams for 1 week.

2. If you start losing weight again, then raise it by 5 grams for one week. If weight loss resumes, continue increasing your allowance by 5 grams every week until it stops. That is your personal carb balance. You'll stick to this number indefinitely, checking your weight every month to make sure you stay at the same weight.

Phase 3 will prepare you for your new lifestyle. By the time you finish this step, you'll be eating somewhere around 80 to 100 carbs per day. You'll find that your diet is nowhere near as restrictive as it once was. Just remember that you need to stay away from wasted carbohydrates like sodas and chips. Stick with healthier options.

Step 4: Make a Lifetime Commitment

All of the hard work is over. Your weight is at an optimal level and you've never had more energy. You've adjusted your body so that it's using carbs more quickly and still burning fat. While you are allowed to eat most healthy carbs like brown rice or whole wheat bread, you should never go above 100 grams per day. For instance, if you decide to have pancakes for breakfast, then you should make sure the rest of your day is full of low-carb choices so that it all balances out.

You will need to stay motivated too, which is what will make up the majority of this phase. That will be the perfect segue to the next chapter of this book.

Chapter 6
Exercising While on the Atkins Diet

Millions of people are starting their journey to a healthier lifestyle by decreasing the number of carbs they consume. Low-carb dieting is definitely the popular choice today and for good reason! It works and makes us feel amazing. However, if you are an avid proponent of exercise and start on this journey, you will probably experience some side effects in the beginning. You'll be more sore than usual after an intense workout and you will also get fatigued more quickly.

Simply put, your body depends on carbohydrates for energy during intense training. This is a downside of the Atkins diet and we have to adapt to it. It's worth noting that these symptoms only occur in the beginning. Once your body learns how to burn fat as a primary source of fuel, then you will be able to train harder.

Strength Training on the Atkins Diet

Okay, so low-carb dieting is going to lower your body fat level even though you'll be eating mostly fatty foods. That's a very difficult concept to grasp, but there is science behind it. The problem is that losing this weight will also mean sacrificing some of your lean muscle mass. When you have a low store of glucose, your muscles are going to react poorly to extended strength training sessions. You might even suffer a decrease in your strength. Fortunately, there are ways around this. Keep in mind that carb restriction is also only a temporary thing. You will be eating carbs again after a few weeks.

With that said, your body is going to remain in a hypo-caloric state when you're on the Atkins diet. This means that you are taking in fewer calories than you burn. When this happens, your body will constantly be searching for that missing energy. It usually breaks down protein into amino acids which are used for energy. This is why your strength and muscle mass both suffer.

We can structure our exercise routine to compensate for this loss though. You will need to change from long workouts to short, intense workouts. Training volume and intensity have an inverse impact on your body. When following a low-carb diet, you need to go as heavy as possible, as quickly as possible so that the muscle is fresh. Then you will do your high-intensity workout for a very short period of time. This will give you the best results without compromising your muscle mass.

This type of exercise routine is quite intense so you must warm up before each workout to avoid injury. Always begin with a couple of light sets and then move directly into high-intensity workouts. Here's an example of a strength training workout that you can follow:

Exercising While on the Atkins Diet

1. You will start with a major muscle-building workout like curling. Do two short, light warm-up sets of 10-15 reps each and then increase the weight to an amount where you know you'll only be able to do 8 reps at most. Then remove 10% of the weight and do another set of 6 reps. Drop the weight another 10% for your final set and hammer out as many reps as you can until you just can't do it anymore. This entire workout will take 5 minutes.

2. Choose another muscle group and hammer out three hard sets of approximately 8 reps each. The type of workout will depend on the muscles you are trying to work out.

As you can see, the goal is to get in as intense of a workout as possible all fit into a five-minute window. This will push you to the limit and your body will then be allowed to rest. It will strengthen these muscles rather than burn them.

Atkins-Friendly Cardio

This is by far the most powerful type of exercise to combine with the Atkins diet. While you don't have to exercise to lose weight on a low-carb diet, it will provide you with a significant advantage. You will lose nearly twice the weight if you mix in some cardio workouts. Here are some examples. You can choose one of them to suit your lifestyle.

. A 30-minute stationary cycling workout in the morning can provide you with a significant metabolic boost throughout the rest of the day. Have a set-up where you can cycle while catching up on the morning news. Preferably, drink a cup of coffee just before your workout since caffeine can enhance your workout. Do this five days per week.

2. Jog on the treadmill for 15 minutes every day, preferably in the morning. Try to keep your cardio intensity to approximately 70% of your maximum heart rate. You can calculate your heart rate using the following formula:

Max Heart Rate = (220 – Age) 0.7

3. Go for a walk. Rather than being cooped up in your home, try going out for a walk at least once per week. It's therapeutic and will help boost your weight loss efforts. Plus, it motivates you to enjoy your new lifestyle.

The amazing thing about cardio workouts is that your body can learn to fuel them with fat so you will not lose muscle mass. The best time for all cardio is in the morning because it is when our body is most open to exercise. You pretty much set the tone for the rest of the day. You have been fasting as you sleep so this is when you are already burning fat at a high level.

Another amazing effect of combining cardio with the Atkins diet is that it gives you a lot of energy. You won't feel tired like you would with strength training.

Exercising While on the Atkins Diet

One more trick to exercising on a low-carb diet is to strategically plan your carb allowance. You should eat the majority of your carbs immediately after a workout for the best results.

Chapter 7
Stay Motivated to Live a Healthier Life

We all have off days where we fall short and ultimately fail. The key to long-term success is to stay motivated. Setbacks happen. They are not what define our successes or failures but the moment you lose motivation, you have begun down the path of failure. This chapter will walk you through several tips that you can follow to help you stay motivated so that your hard work does not go in vain.

Don't Try Too Hard

One of the keys to long-term success is to keep things as simple as possible. When we try too hard and overcomplicate things, we lose motivation. It becomes confusing and frustrates us. Motivation will become natural. If you find that you have to constantly motivate yourself every day, then you need to identify the problem.

If you happen to feel like your motivation is slipping, then maybe you need to take a few days off from exercising. Or maybe you need to give yourself some kind of reward. The problem with motivation is that the more an individual tries to grab ahold of it, the more agile it becomes. If you put the right plan in place and keep it as simple as possible, then everything else will usually flow naturally. There is no need to overcomplicate anything.

Never Stop Learning About Yourself

Do you need to get the fastest dose of inspiration possible for weight loss? Then learn more about yourself. It is by far the most motivational thing you can do. By fully understanding ourselves, we also understand exactly why we are trying to lose weight in the first place. So when you start to feel the grind, ask yourself these questions:

If I give up now, how will I feel six months from now?

If I give up now, how will it affect my health?

If I give up now, how will my family be affected?

Be Realistic

Don't pin posters of super thin models on your wall as a form of motivation because it will have the opposite effect. There have actually been a handful of studies done regarding this and the results agree. The problem with using these thin models as inspiration is that most of us have very little chance of getting into that kind of shape. A lot of the time, these people are on super strict diets or they have time to exercise for hours a day. They do not represent the majority of people.

Rather than aspire to be like them, learn more about yourself and set goals that will improve your life. Post pictures of your progress. Pin up posters of inspirational quotes. Use daily affirmations as motivation. There are just so many options available to you that you do not need to compare yourself to a model.

Focus on Specific Feelings

Sometimes we can become obsessed with an arbitrary number on a scale. It becomes a point of frustration and will cause us to lose motivation. That's why I told you to base your goals around processes rather than a number. Focus on your mood after you have eaten a healthy meal. Consider how much energy you have after an amazing workout. Weight loss motivation is not found on a scale. It's found in the way it makes you feel.

For instance, if you focus on how much better you feel after eating a healthy meal, then it reinforces just how positive of a change you have made. This will increase your motivation.

Lay Out a Plan

All successful ventures start with a well-defined plan. This will describe every step that must be taken and also has a way of measuring your success. You should treat your health goals as you would a business plan. If you were trying to start a project for a client, then you would not go in blind. You would have a well-laid-out plan of action. We already know how to lay out a plan, but I want you to understand that you must follow through with it if you want to stay motivated through the long term.

Start Acting Healthier

The way we act ultimately shapes what we believe, so you should start acting as if you are leading a healthier life as soon as you begin the Atkins diet. Do not wait until you "lose weight" to follow your ambitions. Start right away! Starting on the Atkins diet is a new way of life. You need to treat it as such. Why would you put off your new and improved lifestyle until you achieve some arbitrary number on a scale?

Hang Inspiration Near the Mirror

Are you trying to lose weight before summer so you can fit into that new swimsuit? Then try hanging it near the mirror so that it can serve as daily inspiration. Visualize yourself wearing it so that you are motivated to keep moving forward. Since you already own the item, this is not some unrealistic goal that you have set for yourself. It's very achievable and it will motivate you to keep pushing yourself.

Imagine Your Life if You Fail

Sure, envisioning yourself wearing that new swimsuit is quite motivational, but sometimes it can be just as motivational to envision your life if you were to fail. Ask yourself, "What will my life be like in five years if I do not stick to this plan?"

Sometimes fear can be the most powerful motivational tool at our disposal. Imagine how bad it could potentially be if you're still overweight five years from now. You'll be at risk for heart disease. You will find yourself still lacking energy. The key here is to be absolutely honest with yourself. Do not sugarcoat it.

Uncover your Motivation to Exercise

You need to uncover your motivation for exercise in order to stay on the right track. The moment it starts to feel like work, you'll increase your chances of skipping it. What inspires you to get healthier?

> ➤ Does your family inspire you? Do you want to make sure that you're around for your kids as they grow up?
> ➤ Are you looking to gain more energy so that you can be more productive?

There are so many factors that might motivate us that it's impossible to review them all. If you want to change your behavior, then you will need to identify patterns and then uncover why they exist. Once you start making these changes, your goals will seem much more compelling.

Stop Weighing Success on a Scale

A scale is definitely a helpful tool for measuring your success, but you should not fall into the trap of weighing yourself every day. I recommend that you only check your weight every two weeks. Put the scale away so that you're not tempted to step on it. When you check your weight loss on a daily basis, it's much more difficult to see your progress. You will lose motivation and freak out over the slightest increase. Your weight will fluctuate from day to day.

Take Daily Photos

A picture is worth a thousand words, so it's really powerful to see pictures as you progress along your weight-loss journey. Build a motivational weight-loss gallery! Track your progress by creating a log that literally shows your weight loss over time. Consider posting these pictures on social media. When you commit to a new lifestyle publicly, you have a much higher chance of success. Being able to actually see the results of your diet is one of the most motivational tools you can possess.

Surround Yourself with Healthy Foods

I cannot tell you the number of clients who have fallen off the wagon because they kept junk food around their home and eventually gave in to their temptation. Stock your kitchen with healthy foods while getting rid of all unhealthy choices. You can also decorate your kitchen with beautiful fruit bowls. There are so many steps you can take to motivate yourself into staying on top of your new lifestyle.

Use Technology to Your Advantage

There are thousands of weight loss apps available for your smartphone so you can quite literally pull motivation out of your pocket. I mean, there is an exercise app called "Zombies, Run" where you are running from zombies in a game of survival. My point is that motivation is not too difficult to find in today's world.

Face Your Fears Early

It might not be your lack of motivation but fears that are keeping you from reaching your goals. If you find yourself struggling to stick to your plan, then you need to uncover the underlying reason. Why do you keep failing? A lot of the time, we discover hidden fears that are buried deep within us. For instance, some people worry about what others might think about their new diet. Or they are too embarrassed to exercise in front of other people. Whatever the case, you need to face these fears early. Share your new dieting plan on Facebook. Pair with a friend for your gym visits. Just remember that you're going to receive unsolicited advice from people you barely know.

Chapter 8
Continued Success on the Atkins Diet

As you begin your journey to a healthier lifestyle, you are going to come up against adversity. Whether it's cravings, cookies, or a nice hot slice of pizza, you will struggle in the beginning. If it were easy, then the world would not be facing an obesity pandemic. The problem with giving in is that failure has a snowball effect. One candy bar is not going to thwart your goals at all, but continuous cheating will. Carbs are a rollercoaster ride of ups and downs. You will have cravings in the beginning, but as long as you stick with your plan, then those cravings will go away. I feel that the best way to end this book is to show you some tips that will help you find continued success on the Atkins diet.

Tip #1: Understand How it Works

I want you to read this book again and really pay attention to the science behind the Atkins diet. You must understand how it works so that you can make better decisions. You will learn how certain foods affect your body so that knowledge will help you maintain your weight-loss goals. When you start creating recipes, this information becomes invaluable. Finally, when you understand the science behind low-carb dieting, you will be able to understand food labels.

Tip #2: Never Stop Tracking Carbs

You should never stop counting carbs, even when you are on Phase 4 of the Atkins diet. This is where keeping a food journal really comes in handy. You should always keep your diet under 100 grams of carbs. It's so easy to lose track in the world we live in. While going over one day is not going to hurt, you might quickly find yourself breaking that 100-gram mark every day if you're not keeping track.

Tip #3: Be Sensible about Portion Sizes

You need to be sensible without obsessing about portion sizes. There are actually ways to do this with very little effort. For instance, replace your standard plates with smaller ones. Always wait at least 15 minutes before going back for seconds. In most cases, you'll find that you won't even want seconds after 15 minutes. You should be tracking your calories to make sure you're getting enough. Believe it or not, I've known people whose appetite became so suppressed that they ended up not eating enough calories. This actually resulted in a significant metabolic loss.

Tip #4: Never Allow Yourself to go Hungry

I know! A diet where you are told to never go hungry is not how we've been raised, but the truth is that you should always eat when you're hungry. What's important is that you eat healthy. Have snacks readily available. A palm full of nuts or seeds, or even a small piece of fruit, would be an amazing snack choice.

Tip #5: Protein Should be Included with Every Meal

Always include protein with every meal. You should eat at least 4 ounces with every major meal. Eggs or meat work fine but you will need to make sure that your meal has enough fat so that your body remains in ketosis. You can even have bacon for breakfast. In fact, bacon would be an amazing choice since it's high in fat. Just be sure that you don't choose bacon that is cured using sugar. Another trick is to cook your meats in butter or olive oil.

Tip #6: Savor Fatty Foods

Avocados are one of the healthiest foods on the planet but they are loaded in fat. Fat is the key to being successful on the Atkins diet. Just be sure that the majority of your fats are healthy ones. Trans fat is the only one you should avoid altogether since it's manufactured in processed meals. Every other fat can be a healthy part of the Atkins diet.

Tip #7: Avoid Added Sugar

Even though you can consume 100 grams of carbs once you reach the pinnacle of your Atkins diet journey, you should always stay away from any foods that contain added sugar. For instance, sodas should be permanently given up. You can indulge in the occasional diet soda as long as you don't overdo it. Never should you exceed two diet drinks in a day. Also, remember that artificial sweeteners will lead to sugar cravings so it's best to stay away from them most of the time. Stick to foods that contain natural sugar, like fruits.

Tip #8: Eat Plenty of Vegetables

Once you get to Phase 4 of the Atkins diet, you should be consuming at least 15 grams of carbohydrates per day in the form of vegetables. You will be meeting your daily goal of vegetables while getting plenty of fiber. Vegetables make you feel amazing, so eat plenty. I find that the majority of my meals are vegetable based with added fat and a small portion of protein. But you can choose meatier options as long as you're getting your 15 grams of carbs from vegetables.

Tip #9: You Can Still Eat Out

Unlike other dieting programs, you are able to eat out while following the Atkins diet since it's so flexible. Just pay attention to the menu and replace unhealthy foods with healthier choices. It doesn't take long to learn what foods you can eat and which ones you should avoid. While I usually encourage my clients to avoid fast food, you can occasionally indulge as long as you stick to the low-carb section of the menu.

Tip #10: Take Supplements

Supplements are an amazing way to enhance any diet because we sometimes lack certain nutrients. However, a multivitamin will fill in the gaps. You just have to be sure that you are taking them in conjunction with a healthy diet, not in the place of it.

Some people will take supplements so that they can make unhealthy choices without the guilt. I don't care what they claim, you cannot lose weight unless you clean up your eating habits. No amount of supplements will change that fact!

Tip #11: Measure Your Success
Track your successes so that you have a motivational tool right in front of you! This is not just about pounds, but keep pictures of yourself through the entire process so you can visually see the changes. You can even measure your waist every couple of weeks so that you have another reference to motivate you. This is one of the reasons why keeping a food journal helps you find success.

If you follow these tips, you will be much more likely to achieve long-term success.

Final Thoughts

Does it work?

That's the million-dollar question, and research has shown that low-carb diets like the Atkins diet will help you transform your body into a fat-burning machine. If you are like most others, then you are filling up on processed carbs like breads and pasta. But you are not eating as many fruits and veggies as you should be. The whole point of the Atkins diet is to clean up the damage caused by the traditional Western diet while helping you develop better eating habits.

This book has laid the groundwork for you to get started on this healthier lifestyle, but you are going to have to change the way you look at food. Remember that your health is determined by what you are putting into your body so you need to be sure that what goes in is fueling it in the right way. By the time you are finished with the Atkins diet, you'll be putting much healthier foods into your body.

As you get closer to your weight loss goal, you'll open up the menu of potential foods allowed. The fact is that a low-carb diet is almost impossible to sustain over the long term, so we're just looking to make ourselves conscious of our eating habits so that we can keep it under control. You'll be using this knowledge to shed the pounds when you are overweight and then gradually work healthy carbs back into your diet to

Continued Success on the Atkins Diet

maintain that weight loss. It's designed to be a long-term solution.

One of the important lessons that I hope you have taken away from this book is that fat is not unhealthy. It has gotten a bad reputation but, over the years, nutritional experts have begun to slowly shift the blame away from fats and more towards unhealthy carbs from sugars and processed foods.

As you move forward with your journey to a healthier life, you'll notice that the Atkins diet feels quite restrictive, but your menu will open up as you get close to achieving your weight-loss goals.

Recipes

List of Recipes

Atkins Diet Phase 1 Recipes

Guidelines

During Phase 1 of the Atkins diet, your diet will be based on high-fat, high-protein, and low-carb foods. This is what kick-starts your weight-loss efforts. In essence, you are changing your body into a fat-burning machine. Here are some of the rules that you need to follow:

> ➢ Eat at least 3 meals per day.
> ➢ Never skip a meal and do not go longer than 6 hours without eating. The exception is while you're sleeping.
> ➢ Never eat more than 20 grams of carbohydrates in a day.
> ➢ Most carbs will come from vegetables.
> ➢ Drink at least 8 glasses of water every day.

You need to distinguish hunger from habit during this phase. In short, we mostly eat based on habit so you will find that your appetite is not what makes you overeat.

Always wait 15 minutes before going back for seconds. Most of the time, you will find that you are satisfied. You just need to wait for the food to catch up.

Almond Garlic Crackers

Ingredients

- ✓ ½ cup almond meal
- ✓ ½ cup ground flaxseed
- ✓ ½ cup water
- ✓ 1/3 cup shredded Parmesan cheese
- ✓ 1 tsp. garlic powder
- ✓ ½ tsp. sea salt

Directions

1. Preheat oven to 400 degrees. Line a baking sheet with parchment paper.

2. Mix together almond meal, ground flaxseed, water, Parmesan cheese, garlic powder, and salt in a large bowl. Place to the side until the water has been absorbed, approximately 5 minutes. The dough should easily hold together at this point.

3. Place the dough onto a baking sheet and top it with wax paper. Flatten dough to 1/8 of an inch using either your hands or a rolling pin. Remove wax paper.

4. Make indentations with a knife where you plan to separate into crackers. Then bake at 400 degrees for approximately 15 minutes. It should turn a golden brown color.

5. Remove crackers and allow them to cool for 30 minutes before breaking them into individual crackers.

Recipes

Nutritional Information (per serving)

Total Servings: 8

Calories: 72

Fat: 6g

Carbs: 3g

Fiber: 2.3g

Protein: 3g

Cholesterol: 2mg

Baked Eggs with Cheesy Hash

Ingredients

- ✓ 5 oz. diced zucchini
- ✓ 6 oz. chopped cauliflower
- ✓ ½ red bell pepper, medium and diced
- ✓ 1 tbsp. melted coconut oil
- ✓ 1 tsp. smoked paprika
- ✓ 1 tsp. onion powder
- ✓ 1 tsp. garlic powder
- ✓ ¼ cup Mexican blend shredded cheese
- ✓ ½ avocado, medium
- ✓ 3 large eggs
- ✓ 1 tbsp. sliced jalapenos

- ✓ 3 tbsp. cotija cheese
- ✓ 2 tsp. Tajin seasoning

Instructions

1. Preheat oven to 400 degrees.

2. Line a baking sheet with foil and spread zucchini, cauliflower, and red peppers evenly onto baking pan. Then drizzle it with oil.

3. Sprinkle onion powder, garlic, and paprika, and then toss it all so that the seasonings blend into the mixture.

4. Bake for 15 minutes until it starts to brown.

5. Remove the vegetables from oven and then top with shredded Mexican cheese.

6. Place the avocados around the veggies and crack 3 eggs so that they fill the spaces in between. Bake for approximately 10 minutes. Then add cotija cheese, jalapenos (optional), and Tajin on top of eggs.

Nutritional Information (per serving)

Total Servings: 3

Calories: 248

Fat: 18g

Carbs: 6g

Fiber: 0.2g

Protein: 12g

Cholesterol: 351mg

Breakfast Roll-Ups

Ingredients

- ✓ 10 large eggs
- ✓ Dash of sea salt
- ✓ Dash of ground black pepper
- ✓ 1 ½ cups cheddar cheese, shredded
- ✓ 5 slices cooked bacon
- ✓ 5 cooked breakfast sausage patties
- ✓ Nonstick cooking spray

Instructions

1. Whisk 2 eggs in a bowl and then cook them in a skillet on medium heat. You should spray the skillet with nonstick cooking spray before placing eggs into it. Season these eggs with sea salt and pepper. Cover skillet while eggs thoroughly cook.

. Sprinkle 1/3 cup of cheese on the eggs. Lay down one strip f bacon, and then top that with a sausage patty. You will then need to carefully fold the egg until it looks like a breakfast burrito.

3. Repeat this until you have 5 breakfast rolls.

Nutritional Information (per serving)

Total Servings: 5

Calories: 412

Fat: 31g

Carbs: 2g

Fiber: 0.5g

Protein: 28g

Cholesterol: 20mg

Broccoli and Chicken Casserole

- ✓ 2 heads of broccoli cut into florets (you can use frozen if you wish)
- ✓ 1 large rotisserie chicken, separated from bone
- ✓ 1 cup mayonnaise
- ✓ 2/3 cup whipping cream, heavy
- ✓ 1 tbsp. chicken soup base
- ✓ 1 tbsp. dried dill weed
- ✓ 1 tsp. ground black pepper

- ✓ 2 cups cheddar cheese, shredded
- ✓ Cooking spray

Instructions

1. Preheat oven to 350 degrees.

2. Place broccoli florets into a baking pan. Sprinkle cheese on top and then press down on the broccoli.

3. Mix mayonnaise, chicken soup base, dill, pepper, and heavy cream. Spread this mixture over the chicken and sprinkle shredded cheese on top of it. Place chicken into baking pan.

4. Coat a piece of aluminum foil with the cooking spray and then cover the baking sheet, making sure the greased side is down.

5. Place baking pan in oven for approximately 45 minutes. Then remove aluminum foil and continue baking for 15 minutes. Remove from oven.

6. Let casserole stand for at least 10 minutes.

Nutritional Information (per serving)

Total Servings: 8

Calories: 335

Fat: 22g

Carbs: 6g

Fiber: 3.5g

Protein: 17g

Cholesterol: 99mg

Chicken Lettuce Wraps

Ingredients

- ✓ 1 chicken, deli roasted with meat removed and shredded
- ✓ ½ cup shredded carrots
- ✓ ½ cup water chestnuts
- ✓ 1/3 cup salad dressing, Asian style
- ✓ ¼ cup Greek yogurt
- ✓ 1 pinch of red pepper flakes
- ✓ 1 head of Boston lettuce leaves

Directions

1. Mix together carrots, chicken, and water chestnuts.

2. Mix together salad dressing and yogurt in a separate bowl. It will become a smooth mixture. Pour it over the chicken, then mix and toss it all together.

3. Spoon this newly created mixture into the lettuce leaves. Season with red pepper flakes.

Recipes

Nutritional Information (per serving)

Total Servings: 8

Calories: 362

Fat: 25g

Carbs: 8g

Fiber: 1g

Protein: 27g

Cholesterol: 356mg

Chicken-Stuffed Avocado

Ingredients

- ✓ 4 halved avocados
- ✓ 2 chicken breasts, cooked and shredded
- ✓ 4 oz. cream cheese
- ✓ ¼ cup tomatoes, chopped
- ✓ ¼ tsp. sea salt
- ✓ ¼ tsp. black pepper
- ✓ 1 pinch of cayenne pepper
- ✓ ½ cup shredded Parmesan cheese

Directions

. Preheat oven to 400 degrees.

2. Scoop out the flesh inside of the avocado and place it into a bowl. Add chicken, cream cheese, tomatoes, salt, pepper, and cayenne pepper to the bowl and mix together. You will then scoop this mixture back into the avocado wells. Top with Parmesan cheese.

3. Place avocado halves face up in a muffin pan to keep them upright and bake at 400 degrees for 10 minutes.

Nutritional Information (per serving)

Total Servings: 8

Calories: 334

Fat: 25g

Carbs: 9g

Fiber: 6.8g

Protein: 20g

Cholesterol: 61mg

Laura's Breadless Fried Egg Sandwich

Ingredients

- ✓ 3 slices of bacon
- ✓ 2 eggs
- ✓ Dash of sea salt

- ✓ Dash of black pepper
- ✓ 1/3 cup cheddar cheese, shredded

Directions

1. Place slices of bacon into a large skillet and cook on medium, turning occasionally until crispy. This will take approximately 10 minutes. Drain these slices and place onto paper towels to remove grease. Then crumble the bacon into pieces.

2. In another skillet, crack eggs and season with salt and pepper. Cook until egg whites are firm. This will take approximately 4 minutes. Flip and finish cooking. Sprinkle bacon pieces over one egg and cheese. Cook until cheese has melted. Place second egg on top to create a sandwich.

Nutritional Information (per serving)

Total Servings: 1

Calories: 477

Fat: 38g

Carbs: 2g

Fiber: 34g

Protein: 29g

Cholesterol: 91mg

Spinach Quiche

Ingredients

- ✓ 10 oz. package of frozen spinach, chopped and thawed
- ✓ 1 bunch of green onions finely chopped
- ✓ 4 eggs, beaten
- ✓ 16 oz. package of cottage cheese
- ✓ 2 cups cheddar cheese, shredded
- ✓ ¼ cup crushed croutons

Directions

1. Preheat oven to 325 degrees. Grease a pie pan with olive oil.

2. Place the spinach into a small saucepan and cook on medium until it's soft. This only takes a few minutes. Drain away any liquid that happens to remain.

3. Add green onions, eggs, cottage cheese, and cheddar cheese to the saucepan and stir together. Pour this mixture into the greased pie pan.

4. Bake at 325 degrees for 45 minutes and then remove from heat. Sprinkle with crushed croutons and return to oven for another 15 minutes.

Nutritional Information (per serving)

Total Servings: 4

Calories: 231

Fat: 15g

Carbs: 6g

Fiber: 1.8g

Protein: 19g

Cholesterol: 131mg

Tilapia Parmesan

Ingredients

- ✓ ½ cup Parmesan cheese
- ✓ ¼ cup butter, softened
- ✓ 3 tbsp. mayonnaise
- ✓ 2 tbsp. lemon juice
- ✓ ¼ tsp. dried basil
- ✓ ¼ tsp. black pepper
- ✓ 1/8 tsp. onion powder
- ✓ 1/8 tsp. celery salt
- ✓ 2 lb. tilapia fillets

Directions

1. Preheat oven broiler and then line a baking pan with aluminum foil.

2. Mix together Parmesan cheese, butter, mayonnaise, and lemon juice in a bowl. Then season with dried basil, pepper, onion powder, and celery salt. Mix again to make sure it's all well blended.

3. Place fillets into the baking pan. You should broil them a few inches from the heat for 3 minutes and then flip them, broiling for 2 more minutes. Remove fillets from oven.

4. Coat fillets with cheese mixture and broil for 2 more minutes until the topping is brown.

Nutritional Information (per serving)

Total Servings: 8

Calories: 224

Fat: 13g

Carbs: 1g

Fiber: 0.1g

Protein: 25g

Cholesterol: 63mg

Zucchini Nachos

Ingredients

- ✓ 2 medium-sized zucchini
- ✓ 1 tbsp. olive oil
- ✓ ½ tsp. sea salt
- ✓ ½ finely chopped medium onion
- ✓ 1 lb. ground chicken or turkey
- ✓ 1 tsp. chili powder
- ✓ ½ tsp. paprika
- ✓ ½ tsp. cumin
- ✓ ½ tsp. garlic powder
- ✓ ½ tsp. oregano
- ✓ ¼ tsp. black pepper
- ✓ 2 cups shredded cheese
- ✓ ½ cup low-fat sour cream
- ✓ ½ cup Pico de Gallo
- ✓ 1 sliced jalapeno pepper
- ✓ 3 chopped green onions

Directions

1. Cut zucchini into smaller slices (1/4 inch) and then place them into a colander. Sprinkle with sea salt and then toss in order to coat. Allow it to drain for 30 minutes and then place the slices onto a kitchen towel to pat dry.

2. Preheat oven to 400 degrees and line a baking sheet with parchment paper.

3. In a skillet, heat oil and add onions and sauté until translucent. This will take approximately 2-3 minutes. Add the chicken and cook until it is light brown. Break the meat into small crumbles and cook for approximately 5 minutes. Drain any liquid that accumulates.

4. Reduce skillet to low heat and mix in chili powder, paprika, cumin, garlic powder, salt, oregano, and black pepper. Make sure that you keep this mixture warm.

5. Place zucchini slices into the baking pan and bake at 400 degrees for 5 minutes.

6. Remove zucchini from the oven and top slices with the chicken mixture and cheese. Return to oven and bake for another 2 minutes, until the cheese has melted.

7. Top the nachos with sour cream, Pico de Gallo, jalapeno, and green onions.

Nutritional Information (per serving)

Total Servings: 8

Calories: 311

Fat: 18g

Carbs: 6g

Fiber: 1.4g

Protein: 29g

Cholesterol: 91mg

Atkins Diet Phase 2 Recipes

Guidelines

You will slowly be adding in more carbs to your diet. This must be done slowly so that your body can adapt. Nuts and fruits are the best carbs to start with. As you slowly add carbs into your diet, you will start to understand your body better. You are still going to be losing weight, but the speed will decrease a bit as you add more carbs.

- ➢ Start consuming 30 grams of carbs per day and add an extra 5 grams per week. Stop at 40 grams and remain there for 2 weeks before moving on.
- ➢ Continue to monitor your weight and carb intake. If you stop losing weight, then lower your carb intake by 5 grams.
- ➢ Continue to eat plenty of fats and protein.
- ➢ Drink 8 glasses of water per day.

Famous Butter Chicken

Ingredients

- ✓ 2 eggs, beaten
- ✓ 1 cup crushed buttery round cracker crumbs
- ✓ ½ tsp. garlic salt
- ✓ Dash of black pepper
- ✓ 4 boneless, skinless chicken breasts
- ✓ ½ cup butter, cut into pieces

Directions

1. Preheat oven to 375 degrees.

2. Place eggs and cracker crumbs into separate bowls. Mix garlic salt and pepper with cracker crumbs. Dip chicken into the eggs and then coat them with the crumb mix.

3. Arrange the chicken in a baking pan and place pieces of butter around the chicken.

4. Bake chicken at 375 degrees for 40 minutes. It will no longer be pink in the center.

Nutritional Information (per serving)

Total Servings: 8

Calories: 448

Fat: 31g

Carbs: 9g

Fiber: 0.4g

Protein: 32g

Cholesterol: 222mg

Garlic Chicken

Ingredients

- ✓ ¼ cup olive oil
- ✓ 2 cloves of crushed garlic
- ✓ ¼ cup Italian-seasoned bread crumbs
- ✓ ¼ cup grated Parmesan cheese
- ✓ 4 skinless and boneless chicken breasts

Directions

1. Preheat oven to 425 degrees.

2. Heat olive oil and garlic in a small saucepan on low until it is warm. This will take approximately 2 minutes. Then transfer this oil/garlic mixture to a shallow bowl.

3. Mix together bread crumbs and cheese in another bowl.

4. Dip the chicken into the oil mixture and then transfer it to the crumb mixture, coating the chicken. Place breaded chicken into a baking dish.

5. Bake at 425 degrees for 35 minutes. The center of the chicken should measure at 165 degrees with a meat thermometer.

Nutritional Information (per serving)

Total Servings: 4

Calories: 300

Fat: 17g

Carbs: 6g

Fiber: 0.3g

Protein: 30g

Cholesterol: 73mg

Homemade Guacamole

Ingredients

- ✓ 3 avocados, peeled and mashed
- ✓ 1 juiced lime
- ✓ 1 tsp. sea salt
- ✓ ½ cup onion, diced
- ✓ 3 tbsp. fresh cilantro, chopped
- ✓ 2 diced Roma tomatoes
- ✓ 1 tsp. minced garlic
- ✓ 1 pinch of ground cayenne pepper

Directions

1. Mash together the avocado, lime juice and salt in a bowl.
2. Then add in onion, cilantro, tomatoes, and garlic. Stir in the cayenne pepper before refrigerating for one hour.

Nutritional Information (per serving)

Total Servings: 6

Calories: 262

Fat: 22g

Carbs: 18g

Fiber: 11g

Protein: 4g

Cholesterol: 596mg

Low-Carb Breakfast Pizza

Ingredients

- ✓ 1 ½ tbsp. butter
- ✓ 6 eggs
- ✓ ¼ cup heavy whipping cream
- ✓ ¼ cup cheddar cheese, shredded
- ✓ ½ cup green bell pepper, chopped
- ✓ 3 slices of bacon

- ✓ ¼ cup chopped onion
- ✓ 3 slices of bacon
- ✓ 2 sausage links, sliced into pepperoni-sized pieces
- ✓ 1/3 cup tomato puree
- ✓ ¼ tsp. garlic powder
- ✓ ¼ tsp. onion powder
- ✓ 1/8 tsp. dried oregano
- ✓ 1/8 tsp. dried basil
- ✓ Dash of sea salt
- ✓ Dash of pepper
- ✓ ¾ cup mozzarella cheese, shredded

Directions

1. Preheat oven to 400 degrees.

2. Heat 1 tbsp. butter in a glass container until it has melted. Then whisk together melted butter, eggs, cream, and cheddar cheese in a large bowl. Pour egg mixture into a pie pan.

3. Bake at 400 degrees for approximately 20 minutes. Remove this egg "crust" from the oven.

4. Melt the rest of the butter in a skillet on medium. Add in onion and green bell pepper. Cook for 5 minutes. Place bacon into the skillet and cook for 10 minutes, until crisp. Then cook the sausage in the same skillet. Drain skillet.

5. Mix together tomato puree, garlic powder, onion power, oregano, basil, salt, and black pepper in a small bowl. This will create the pizza sauce.

6. Top the egg crust with the pizza sauce, cheese, onion and green pepper mixture, bacon, and sausage.

7. Bake pizza at 400 for 10 minutes.

Nutritional Information (per serving)

Total Servings: 8

Calories: 431

Fat: 34g

Carbs: 7g

Fiber: 1g

Protein: 25g

Cholesterol: 356 mg

Marinated Grilled Shrimp

Ingredients

- ✓ 3 cloves of minced garlic
- ✓ 1/3 cup olive oil
- ✓ ¼ cup tomato sauce

Recipes

- ✓ 2 tbsp. red wine vinegar
- ✓ 2 tbsp. fresh basil, chopped
- ✓ ½ tsp. sea salt
- ✓ ¼ tsp. cayenne pepper
- ✓ 2 lbs. fresh shrimp, deveined and peeled

Directions

1. Mix together garlic, olive oil, tomato sauce, and red wine vinegar in a large bowl. Then season this mixture with basil, sea salt, and cayenne pepper. Finally, add shrimp and stir together until it's evenly coated. Cover and refrigerate for one hour, stirring once.

2. Preheat grill to medium and thread shrimp onto skewers.

3. Oil grill grate and grill shrimp skewers for 3 minutes per side.

Nutritional Information (per serving)

Total Servings: 8

Calories: 448

Fat: 31g

Carbs: 9g

Fiber: 0.4g

Protein: 32g

Cholesterol: 222mg

Rempel Family Meatloaf

Ingredients

- ✓ 1 ½ lb. ground beef
- ✓ ½ cup crushed buttery crackers
- ✓ ¾ cup shredded cheddar cheese
- ✓ 1 oz. package of dry onion soup mix
- ✓ 2 eggs, beaten
- ✓ ¼ cup ketchup
- ✓ 2 tbsp. steak sauce

Directions

1. Preheat oven to 350 degrees.

2. Mix together ground beef, crushed crackers, cheddar cheese, and onion soup mix in a large bowl. Whisk the eggs, ketchup, and steak sauce in a separate bowl until smooth. Add in a small touch of water and then press this mixture into a baking loaf pan.

3. Bake in oven at 350 degrees for one hour. The loaf will no longer be pink in the middle.

Nutritional Information (per serving)

Total Servings: 5

Calories: 360

Fat: 23g

Carbs: 9g

Fiber: 0.5g

Protein: 27g

Cholesterol: 143mg

Rosemary Chicken Kabobs

Ingredients

- ✓ ½ cup olive oil
- ✓ ½ cup Ranch dressing
- ✓ 3 tbsp. Worcestershire sauce
- ✓ 1 tbsp. minced fresh rosemary
- ✓ 2 tsp. sea salt
- ✓ ¼ tsp. black pepper
- ✓ 1 tsp. lemon juice
- ✓ 1 tsp. white vinegar
- ✓ 1 tbsp. white sugar
- ✓ 3 skinless, boneless chicken breasts cut into cubes

Directions

. Mix together olive oil, Ranch dressing, Worcestershire sauce, rosemary, salt, lemon juice, white vinegar, pepper, and sugar in a small bowl and allow to stand for approximately 5 minutes.

2. Place the chicken breasts into the bowl with the mixture and coat them. Cover and refrigerate for approximately 1 hour.

3. Preheat your grill on medium and thread chicken cubes onto skewers.

4. Oil the grill grating lightly and then grill skewers for approximately 10 minutes. The chicken will no longer be pink in the center.

Nutritional Information (per serving)

Total Servings: 6

Calories: 378

Fat: 31g

Carbs: 5g

Fiber: 0.1g

Protein: 20g

Cholesterol: 59mg

Rotisserie-Style Chicken

Ingredients

- ✓ 4 tsp. sea salt

Recipes

- ✓ 2 tsp. paprika
- ✓ 1 tsp. onion powder
- ✓ 1 tsp. dried thyme
- ✓ 1 tsp. white pepper
- ✓ ½ tsp. cayenne pepper
- ✓ ½ tsp. black pepper
- ✓ ½ tsp. garlic powder
- ✓ 2 onions cut into quarters
- ✓ 2 whole chickens (4 lb. each)

Directions

1. Mix together sea salt, paprika, onion powder, thyme, white pepper, black pepper, cayenne pepper, and garlic powder in a bowl.

2. Rinse chickens and remove giblets. Pat them dry using a paper towel. Rub the chickens inside and out using the spice mixture. Place 1 onion into each of the chicken cavities.

3. Place chickens in a plastic sealable bag and refrigerate overnight.

4. Preheat oven to 250 degrees.

5. Place the chickens into a roasting pan and bake them for 5 hours, uncovered. They should measure 180 degrees inside. Allow the chickens to cool before carving.

Nutritional Information (per serving)

Total Servings: 8

Calories: 586

Fat: 34g

Carbs: 4g

Fiber: 1g

Protein: 62g

Cholesterol: 194mg

Atkins Diet Phase 3 Recipes

Guidelines

Now we're going to slow down your weight loss even further since you should be close to your goal by this point. You will need to add 5 grams of daily carbs per week to your diet until your weight loss stops. Then reduce your diet by 5 grams per day and stick to that number for a full month.

You will still be losing weight slightly.

The goal of this phase is to begin the transition to your new long-term lifestyle. It's putting on the finishing touches until you have found your carb tolerance.

Amazingly Healthy Chicken

Ingredients

- ✓ ¼ cup cider vinegar
- ✓ 3 tbsp. prepared coarse-ground mustard
- ✓ 3 cloves peeled and minced garlic
- ✓ 1 juiced lime
- ✓ ½ juiced lemon
- ✓ ½ Cup brown sugar
- ✓ 1 ½ tsp. sea salt
- ✓ Dash ground pepper
- ✓ 6 tbsp. olive oil
- ✓ 3 boneless, skinless chicken breasts cut into halves

Directions

1. Mix together cider vinegar, mustard, garlic, lime juice, lemon juice, brown sugar, salt, and pepper in a large bowl. Whisk in the olive oil and place chicken into the mix. Cover and allow it to marinate overnight.

2. Preheat a grill to high.

3. Oil the grating lightly and place chicken on the grill. Cook for approximately 8 minutes per side.

Nutritional Information (per serving)

Total Servings: 6

Calories: 337

Fat: 22g

Carbs: 22g

Fiber: 1g

Protein: 25g

Cholesterol: 67mg

Bubble 'n' Squeak

Ingredients

Mashed Cauliflower

- ✓ Approximately 300 g. cauliflower florets
- ✓ 2 tbsp. heavy whipping cream
- ✓ 1 tbsp. butter
- ✓ Dash of sea salt
- ✓ Dash of ground black pepper

Bubble 'n' Squeak

- ✓ 3 slices of bacon, diced
- ✓ 1 tbsp. butter
- ✓ ¼ diced onion, medium
- ✓ 50 g. sliced leek

- ✓ 1 stalk sliced green onion
- ✓ 50 g. chopped Brussels sprouts
- ✓ ¼ cup mozzarella, grated
- ✓ ¼ cup Parmesan cheese, grated
- ✓ 2 tbsp. duck fat
- ✓ 1 tsp. minced garlic

Instructions

1. You can either use leftover mashed cauliflower, or place the florets into a bowl along with 1 tbsp. butter and cream. Mix it together and then microwave on high for approximately 4 minutes. Mix thoroughly to avoid drying out the cauliflower.

2. Place in the microwave for 4 more minutes. The cauliflower will now be soft. Season with sea salt and pepper.

3. Use a blender to finish mashing the cauliflower until it's creamy. Add mozzarella while it's still hot.

4. Put the chopped bacon into a pan and cook on medium until it's crispy. Remove bacon and place onto a paper towel.

5. Add 1 tbsp. butter to the bacon fat that's left in the pan. Then mix in garlic and cook it for approximately 60 seconds.

6. Add onion to the pan and sauté for approximately 4 minutes. The onion should be translucent.

7. Add in the chopped leeks and Brussels sprouts. Cook them for approximately 10 minutes, or until soft.

8. Add green onions and cook for an additional minute. Remove from heat and allow the pan to cool.

9. Add bacon to the vegetable mix and then add that new mixture to the mashed cauliflower. Season with sea salt and pepper if needed.

10. After mixing together all of the ingredients, add the duck fat cooked in a pan on medium until it's melted. Then place the egg rings into the pan and sprinkle Parmesan into the rings.

11. Add mashed cauliflower into the rings. Sprinkle more Parmesan onto the top of it.

12. Give the mixture a chance to warm (especially if using leftovers.) Flip over and allow to cook until a crisp crust forms. Be careful that they don't get too hot or the mixture may run. If you find they aren't crisping on the outside, turn up the heat on the pan and press down on them for a minute or so on each side.

Nutritional Information (per serving)

Total Servings: 8

Calories: 332

Fat: 28g

Carbs: 11g

Fiber: 3g

Protein: 11g

Cholesterol: 23mg

Chinese Pork Tenderloin

Ingredients

- ✓ 2 pork tenderloins, approximately 1 ½ pounds each – trimmed
- ✓ 2 tbsp. soy sauce
- ✓ 2 tbsp. hoisin sauce
- ✓ 1 tbsp. sherry
- ✓ 1 tbsp. black bean sauce
- ✓ 1 ½ tsp. minced ginger root
- ✓ ½ tsp. brown sugar
- ✓ 1 clove of garlic
- ✓ ½ tsp. sesame oil
- ✓ 1 pinch of Chinese five-spice powder

Directions

1. Place the tenderloins into a glass baking dish.

2. Whisk together soy sauce, hoisin sauce, sherry, black bean sauce, ginger, sugar, garlic, sesame oil, and five-spice powder in a bowl. Pour this marinade over pork tenderloins. Make sure they are coated on both sides. Cover and refrigerate for no less than 2 hours.

3. Preheat oven to 375 degrees.

4. Bake tenderloins at 375 degrees for 35 minutes. Let them stand for 10 minutes before slicing them diagonally. Make several thin slices.

Nutritional Information (per serving)

Total Servings: 12

Calories: 222

Fat: 6g

Carbs: 5g

Fiber: 0.3g

Protein: 36g

Cholesterol: 98mg

Maple Salmon

Ingredients

- ✓ ¼ cup maple syrup
- ✓ 2 tbsp. soy sauce
- ✓ 1 clove of minced garlic
- ✓ ¼ tsp. garlic salt
- ✓ 1/8 tsp. black pepper
- ✓ 1 lb. salmon

Directions

1. Mix together maple syrup, soy sauce, garlic, garlic salt, and pepper in a small bowl.

2. Place salmon into a glass baking dish and coat with maple syrup mix. Cover the dish and place in the refrigerator for one hour. Turn salmon once.

3. Preheat oven to 400 degrees.

4. Place salmon into oven and bake at 400 degrees for 20 minutes.

Nutritional Information (per serving)

Total Servings: 4

Calories: 265

Fat: 12g

Carbs: 14g

Fiber: 0.1g

Protein: 23g

Cholesterol: 67mg

Spaghetti Squash Lasagna

<u>**Ingredients**</u>

- ✓ 1 spaghetti squash
- ✓ 2 tbsp. olive oil
- ✓ ½ medium diced onion
- ✓ 1 lb. breakfast sausage
- ✓ 1 lb. ground beef
- ✓ 1 tbsp. garlic, minced
- ✓ 24 oz. marinara sauce (make sure it's low carb)
- ✓ 20 oz. whole milk ricotta
- ✓ 2 eggs, large
- ✓ ¾ cup Parmesan cheese, grated
- ✓ 2 tbsp. basil, chopped
- ✓ ½ tsp. sea salt
- ✓ ½ tsp. ground pepper
- ✓ 8 oz. mozzarella cheese, sliced
- ✓ 2 tbsp. parsley, chopped

Instructions

1. Preheat oven to 400 degrees.

2. Split the squash in half lengthwise and remove the seeds. Drizzle it with 1 tbsp. olive oil and sprinkle with salt and pepper.

3. Roast for approximately 45 minutes, or until the squash is tender. It should be easy to shred with a fork. Remove from the skin and place it to the side. Drain away any visible liquid.

4. Heat 1 tbsp. of olive oil in a skillet. Add sausage, beef, onion, and garlic. Cook thoroughly until meat has been fully cooked. Drain away any fat/grease.

5. Add marinara sauce to the meat and bring it to a boil. Then allow it to simmer on low for approximately 15 minutes. It should be thick.

6. Combine the ricotta and Parmesan cheeses, eggs, basil, salt, and pepper in a bowl.

7. Reduce oven heat to 350 degrees and grease a casserole dish. In layers, add one layer of squash to the bottom of the dish. Top squash with ricotta mix. Top ricotta mix with meat sauce. Top meat sauce with a layer of mozzarella cheese.

8. Repeat, adding layers as described above until you are out of mixture.

9. Sprinkle the remaining ¼ cup of Parmesan cheese and parsley on top of the lasagna.

10. Cover with foil and bake for 30 minutes. Then remove foil and bake for an additional 20 minutes. You will need to let the lasagna stand for at least 10 minutes before serving it.

Nutritional Information (per serving)

Total Servings: 10

Calories: 578

Fat: 46g

Carbs: 16g

Fiber: 6g

Protein: 30g

Cholesterol: 27mg

Spinach Chicken

Ingredients

✓ 10 oz. artichoke, chopped (you can use frozen or canned...check label)

- ✓ 10 oz. chopped spinach
- ✓ 4 oz. cream cheese
- ✓ 4 oz. mayonnaise
- ✓ 1 cup Parmesan cheese (separated into ½ cups)
- ✓ 1 cup mozzarella (separated into ½ cups)
- ✓ 3 cloves garlic
- ✓ 1 bag chicken tenderloins
- ✓ Sea salt and pepper to taste

Instructions

1. Preheat oven to 400 degrees.

2. Cut chicken into chunks and place them into a baking pan. Season chicken with sea salt and pepper.

3. Bake chicken for 15 minutes by itself.

4. As chicken cooks, combine spinach, artichokes, garlic, cream cheese, mayonnaise, ½ cup Parmesan, and ½ cup mozzarella. Mix this extremely well.

5. When chicken has baked for 15 minutes, remove it and cover with the spinach/artichoke topping that you just created

6. Reduce oven to 350 degrees and bake chicken for 20 minutes.

7. Remove chicken from oven and sprinkle the remainder of the Parmesan and mozzarella on top of it.

8. Place oven on low broil and place chicken back in oven until the cheese is bubbly.

Nutritional Information (per serving)

Total Servings: 8

Calories: 522

Fat: 33g

Carbs: 10g

Fiber: 4g

Protein: 26g

Cholesterol: 96mg

Turkey Veggie Meatloaf Cups

Ingredients

- ✓ 2 cups zucchini, coarsely chopped
- ✓ 1 ½ cups onion, coarsely chopped
- ✓ 1 red bell pepper, coarsely chopped
- ✓ 1 lb. ground turkey
- ✓ ½ cup uncooked couscous
- ✓ 2 tbsp. Worcestershire sauce

✓ 1 tbsp. Dijon mustard

✓ ½ cup barbecue sauce

Directions

1. Preheat oven to 400 degrees and spray 20 muffin cups with cooking spray.

2. Put zucchini, onions, and red bell pepper into a food processor and pulse a few times until it is finely chopped. You do not want it to be liquefied so make sure you just pulse it.

3. Place vegetables into another bowl and mix with ground turkey, couscous, egg, Worcestershire sauce, and Dijon mustard. Fill each of the prepared cups with this mixture until they are ¾ of the way full. Top each cup with 1 tsp. barbecue sauce.

4. Bake at 400 degrees for about 25 minutes. The internal temperature should measure 160 degrees. Allow to stand for 5 minutes before serving.

Nutritional Information (per serving)

Total Servings: 20

Calories: 119

Fat: 1g

Carbs: 14g

Fiber: 1.2g

Protein: 13g

Cholesterol: 47mg

Turmeric Chicken Stew
Ingredients

- ✓ 2 tbsp. olive oil
- ✓ 2 boneless, skinless chicken breasts cut into cubes
- ✓ 2 sweet potatoes cut into cubes
- ✓ ½ chopped red onion
- ✓ 1 eggplant cut into cubes
- ✓ 2 cloves of garlic, minced
- ✓ 1 tbsp. fresh ginger, minced
- ✓ 2 tsp. ground turmeric
- ✓ ½ cup low-sodium chicken broth

Directions

. Heat olive oil in a large skillet on medium and then add
chicken. Cook until browned, approximately 5 minutes.

.. Add sweet potatoes and onion, cooking for 3 minutes before
adding eggplant, garlic, ginger, and turmeric. Cook for 1
minute. Finally, pour in broth and simmer until the stew has
thickened. This takes approximately 20 minutes.

Nutritional Information (per serving)

Total Servings: 4

Calories: 183

Fat: 6g

Carbs: 24g

Fiber: 5g

Protein: 10g

Cholesterol: 20mg

Atkins Diet Phase 4 Recipes

Guidelines

By this point, you should know your carb tolerance so it's all about tracking your foods so that you maintain the same tolerance. If you gain weight, then reduce your carb intake until you steady off.

Phase 4 is your new lifestyle. It becomes your permanent way of eating and it's going to make sure that you keep that weight off. But you must remain diligent.

You will still be eating full-fat foods but you can add some carbs into your life. In fact, the average person can consume 100 grams of carbs per day and not gain weight.

You might have to make adjustments to your diet if your lifestyle changes. For instance, if you move from an office job to a labor-intensive job, then you will probably need to increase your carb intake.

The overall goal is to maintain a steady weight and make adjustments as necessary.

Carrot Cake Oatmeal

Ingredients

- ✓ 2/3 cup chopped pineapple
- ✓ ½ cup sliced carrot
- ✓ 1 tsp. water
- ✓ 2/3 cup almond milk
- ✓ ½ cup old-fashioned oats
- ✓ ½ tsp. ground cinnamon
- ✓ ½ tsp. ground ginger
- ✓ 1 tbsp. chopped walnuts

Directions

1. Mix together pineapple, carrot, and water in a microwave-safe bowl. Cook for approximately 2 minutes until the carrots are softened.

2. Add in the almond milk, oats, cinnamon, and ginger and cook for 1 minute. Stir and cook for 30 seconds. Stir again. Repeat two more times until the oats are soft and fully cooked. Top with walnuts.

Nutritional Information (per serving)

Total Servings: 1

Calories: 305

Fat: 9g

Carbs: 50g

Fiber: 8g

Protein: 8g

Cholesterol: 111mg

Carrot, Tomato, and Spinach Quinoa Pilaf with Ground Turkey

Ingredients

- ✓ 2 tsp. olive oil
- ✓ 1 cup quinoa
- ✓ Half of an onion, chopped
- ✓ 2 tbsp. chicken-flavored vegetable bouillon
- ✓ 1 tsp. black pepper
- ✓ 1 tsp. ground thyme
- ✓ 1 chopped carrot
- ✓ 1 chopped tomato
- ✓ 1 cup baby spinach
- ✓ 2 tbsp. olive oil
- ✓ 1 lb. ground turkey
- ✓ 14 oz. can of black beans, drained

Directions

1. Heat 2 tablespoons of olive oil in a saucepan on medium. Stir in onion and cook for approximately 5 minutes. Reduce heat to medium-low and add quinoa. Cook for 2 minutes, stirring constantly.

2. Pour water into the saucepan and then add bouillon granules, black pepper, and thyme. Bring to a boil. Reduce heat to low and cover, simmering until the quinoa softens. This will take approximately 5 minutes.

3. Stir carrots into the quinoa mixture and cover again. Simmer for 10 minutes until all of the water has been absorbed.

4. Remove saucepan from heat and mix tomatoes and spinach into the quinoa mixture. The spinach will quickly wilt.

5. Heat the rest of the olive oil in a large skillet and cook turkey on medium. This takes about 7 minutes. Drain grease and mix in black beans with turkey, cooking on medium for approximately 3 minutes to heat up the beans.

6. Add the quinoa mixture until it has been thoroughly heated. This takes approximately 5 minutes.

Nutritional Information (per serving)

Total Servings: 6

Calories: 422

Fat: 17g

Carbs: 41g

Fiber: 9.6g

Protein: 29g

Cholesterol: 67mg

Corned Beef & Cabbage

Ingredients

- ✓ 1 corned beef brisket (approximately 5 ½ lbs.)
- ✓ 2 tbsp. pickling spice
- ✓ 1 sliced orange
- ✓ 2 sliced stalks of celery
- ✓ 1 sliced onion
- ✓ ¾ cup cold water
- ✓ 6 tbsp. butter
- ✓ 1 large head of cabbage, sliced and cored
- ✓ 1 cup apples, sliced and peeled

Directions

. Preheat oven to 300 degrees. Place a sheet of aluminum foil into the bottom of a roasting pan. Make sure to leave enough excess foil so that you can seal the entire roast later.

2. Rub the brisket with the pickling spice and then place it into the pan you just prepared. Place celery, orange, and onion slices evenly around the beef. Add ½ cup of water and then wrap the aluminum foil so that you seal the roast inside of the foil.

3. Bake beef for 3 hours in the oven, or until the meat becomes tender.

4. Approximately 3 hours into cooking the roast, place butter and ¼ cup water into a pot. Add cabbage and apples. Cover and simmer on low for approximately 30 minutes. Shake the pot occasionally so that the cabbage does not stick to the bottom.

5. Serve cabbage and corned beef together.

Nutritional Information (per serving)

Total Servings: 12

Calories: 482

Fat: 34g

Carbs: 26g

Fiber: 9g

Protein: 27g

Cholesterol: 123mg

Healthy Ham Sandwiches

Ingredients

- ✓ 6 lb. ham with the bone
- ✓ 8 oz. jar of yellow mustard
- ✓ 1 lb. brown sugar
- ✓ 24 dinner rolls

Directions

1. Place ham into a slow cooker and cover with water. Cook for 8 hours.

2. Remove the ham from the water and allow it to cool. It should fall to pieces as you pick it up.

3. Once the ham has cooled, pull it into shreds. Place shredded ham into the slow cooker and mix in mustard and brown sugar. Cook on low.

4. Serve ham on dinner rolls. You may use other sandwich toppings if desired.

Nutritional Information (per serving)

Total Servings: 24

Calories: 445

Fat: 23g

Carbs: 34g

Fiber: 1g

Protein: 24g

Cholesterol: 65mg

Roasted Veggies

Ingredients

- ✓ 1 small butternut squash cut into cubes
- ✓ 2 red bell peppers, diced and seeded
- ✓ 1 sweet potato peeled and cut into cubes
- ✓ 3 potatoes cut into cubes
- ✓ 1 red onion cut into quarters
- ✓ 1 tbsp. chopped thyme
- ✓ 2 tbsp. chopped fresh rosemary
- ✓ ¼ cup olive oil
- ✓ 2 tbsp. balsamic vinegar
- ✓ Dash of sea salt
- ✓ Dash of black pepper

Directions

1. Preheat oven to 475 degrees.

2. Mix together squash, red bell peppers, sweet potato, and potatoes. Separate onion into pieces and add them to the mixture.

3. Mix together thyme, rosemary, olive oil, vinegar, salt, and pepper. Toss with the veggies until they are coated. Spread this evenly into a roasting pan.

4. Roast veggies in oven at 475 degrees for 35 minutes, stirring every 10 minutes. The veggies will be tender and thoroughly browned.

Nutritional Information (per serving)

Total Servings: 4

Calories: 123

Fat: 5g

Carbs: 20g

Fiber: 3g

Protein: 2g

Cholesterol: 0mg

Rice Cooker Oats

Ingredients

- ✓ 1 cup quick-cooking oats
- ✓ 1 cup water
- ✓ 1 cup milk
- ✓ 2 tbsp. honey
- ✓ 1 tbsp. sugar
- ✓ 1 tsp. vanilla extract
- ✓ Pinch of sea salt

Directions

1. Mix together oats, water, milk, honey, sugar, vanilla extract, and salt in a rice cooker.

2. Cook oats for approximately up to 15 minutes until it is the consistency you desire.

Nutritional Information (per serving)

Total Servings: 1

Calories: 309

Fat: 5g

Carbs: 57g

Fiber: 4.1g

Protein: 9g

Cholesterol: 135mg

Recipes

Turkey Chili

Ingredients

- ✓ 1 ½ tsp. olive oil
- ✓ 1 lb. ground turkey
- ✓ 1 chopped onion
- ✓ 2 cups water
- ✓ 28 oz. can of crushed tomatoes
- ✓ 16 oz. can of kidney beans, drained and mashed
- ✓ 1 tbsp. minced garlic
- ✓ 2 tbsp. chili powder
- ✓ ½ tsp. paprika
- ✓ ½ tsp. dried oregano
- ✓ ½ tsp. ground cayenne pepper
- ✓ ½ tsp. ground cumin
- ✓ ½ tsp. sea salt
- ✓ ½ tsp. black pepper

Directions

1. Heat oil in a large pot on medium. Place turkey into pot and cook until it's evenly browned. Mix in onion and cook until it's tender.

2. Pour water into the pot and then add tomatoes, kidney beans, and garlic. Season with chili powder, paprika, oregano, cayenne pepper, cumin, salt, and pepper. Bring pot to a boil

and then reduce heat to low, cover, and simmer for 30 minutes.

Nutritional Information (per serving)

Total Servings: 8

Calories: 185

Fat: 6g

Carbs: 19g

Fiber: 6g

Protein: 16g

Cholesterol: 42mg

Un-Refried Beans

Ingredients

- ✓ 1 onion, halved and peeled
- ✓ 2 cups dry pinto beans
- ✓ ½ fresh jalapeno, seeded and chopped
- ✓ 2 tbsp. minced garlic
- ✓ 5 tsp. sea salt
- ✓ ¾ tsp. black pepper
- ✓ 1/8 tsp. ground cumin
- ✓ 9 cups water

Directions

1. Place the onion, beans, jalapeno, garlic, salt, pepper, and cumin into a slow cooker. Pour water and stir to combine all ingredients. Cook on high for 8 hours, adding more water if needed.

2. Once the beans have finished cooking, save the liquid after draining them. Mash the beans with a potato masher and then add reserved water as needed.

Nutritional Information (per serving)

Total Servings: 8

Calories: 139

Fat: 0.5g

Carbs: 25g

Fiber: 6g

Protein: 9g

Cholesterol: 785mg

Conversion Tables

U.S. Standard	U.S. St. Ounces	Metric
2 Tbsp.	1 fl. Oz.	30 mL
1/4 Cup	2 fl. Oz.	60 mL
1/2 Cup	4 fl. Oz.	120 mL
1 Cup	8 fl. Oz.	240 mL
1 ½ Cup	12 fl. Oz.	355 mL
2 Cups	16 fl. Oz.	475 mL
4 Cups	32 fl. Oz.	1 L
1 Gallon	128 fl. Oz.	4 L

Oven Temperatures

Fahrenheit (F)	Celsius (C)
250 F	120 C
300 F	150 C
325 F	165 C
350 F	180 C
375 F	190 C
400 F	200 C
425 F	220 C
450 F	230 C

Recipes

Liquid Volume

Standard U.S.	Metric
1/8 Tsp.	0.5 mL
1/4 Tsp.	1 mL
1/2 Tsp.	2 mL
2/3 Tsp.	4 mL
1 Tsp.	5 mL
1 Tbsp.	15 mL
1/4 Cup	59 mL
1/3 Cup	79 mL
1/2 Cup	118 mL
2/3 Cup	156 mL
3/4 Cup	177 mL
1 Cup	235 mL
2 Cups / 1 Pint	475 mL
3 Cups	700 mL
4 Cups / 1 Quart	1 L
1/2 Gallon	2 L
1 Gallon	4 L

Weight Conversion

U.S. Standard	Metric
1/2 Ounce	15 g
1 Ounce	30 g
2 Ounces	60 g
4 Ounces	115 g
8 Ounces	225 g
12 Ounces	340 g
16 Ounces / 1 Pound	455 g

One Last Thing... Did You Enjoy the Book?

If so, then let me know by leaving a review on Amazon! Reviews are the lifeblood of independent authors. I would appreciate even a few words from you!

If you did not like the book, then please tell me! Email me at lizard.publishing@gmail.com and let me know what you didn't like. Perhaps I can change it. In today's world, a book doesn't have to be stagnant. It should be improved with time and feedback from readers like you. You can impact this book, and I welcome your feedback. Help me make this book better for everyone!

56926819R00090

Made in the USA
Middletown, DE
25 July 2019